Environmental Issues and Allergy

Editor

JILL A. POOLE

IMMUNOLOGY AND ALLERGY CLINICS OF NORTH AMERICA

https://www.immunology.theclinics.com/

November 2022 • Volume 42 • Number 4

ELSEVIER

1600 John F. Kennedy Boulevard • Suite 1800 • Philadelphia, Pennsylvania, 19103-2899

http://www.theclinics.com

IMMUNOLOGY AND ALLERGY CLINICS OF NORTH AMERICA Volume 42, Number 4

November 2022 ISSN 0889-8561, ISBN-13: 978-0-323-96091-5

Editor: Taylor Hayes
Developmental Editor: Jessica Cañaberal

Immunology and Allergy Clinics of North America (ISSN 0889–8561) is published quarterly by Elsevier Inc., 360 Park Avenue South, New York, NY 10010-1710. Months of issue are February, May, August, and November. Periodicals postage paid at New York, NY and additional mailing offices. Subscription prices are $354.00 per year for US individuals, $844.00 per year for US institutions, $100.00 per year for US students and residents, $432.00 per year for Canadian individuals, $100.00 per year for Canadian students, $861.00 per year for Canadian institutions, $456.00 per year for international individuals, $861.00 per year for international institutions, $220.00 per year for international students. To receive student/resident rate, orders must be accompanied by name of affiliated institution, date of term, and the *signature* of program/residency coordinator on institution letterhead. Orders will be billed at individual rate until proof of status is received. Foreign air speed delivery is included in all *Clinics* subscription prices. All prices are subject to change without notice. **POSTMASTER**: Send address changes to *Immunology and Allergy Clinics of North America*, Elsevier Health Sciences Division, Subscription Customer Service, 3251 Riverport Lane, Maryland Heights, MO 63043. **Customer Service: 1-800-654-2452 (U.S. and Canada); 314-447-8871 (outside U.S. and Canada). Fax: 314-447-8029. E-mail: journalscustomerservice-usa@elsevier.com** (for print support); **journalsonlinesupport-usa@elsevier.com** (for online support).

Reprints. For copies of 100 or more, of articles in this publication, please contact the Commercial Reprints Department, Elsevier Inc., 360 Park Avenue South, New York, New York 10010-1710. Tel. 212-633-3874, Fax: 212-633-3820, E-mail: reprints@elsevier.com.

Immunology and Allergy Clinics of North America is covered in MEDLINE/PubMed (Index Medicus), Current Contents/Life Sciences, Science Citation Index, ISI/BIOMED, Chemical Abstracts, and EMBASE/Excerpta Medica.

Contributors

EDITOR

JILL A. POOLE, MD
Professor, Division of Allergy and Immunology, Department of Internal Medicine, College of Medicine, University of Nebraska Medical Center, Omaha, Nebraska

AUTHORS

CLAIRE E. ATKINSON, MD
Fellow-in-Training, Division of Allergy and Immunology, Department of Pediatrics, University of North Carolina School of Medicine, Chapel Hill, North Carolina

TINA M. BANZON, MD
Boston Children's Hospital, Boston, Massachusetts

JONATHAN A. BERNSTEIN, MD
Department of Internal Medicine, Division of Rheumatology, Allergy and Immunology, Professor of Clinical Medicine, University of Cincinnati College of Medicine, Cincinnati, Ohio

CHRISTOPHER D. BROOKS, MD
Allergy/Immunology Fellow, Department of Otolaryngology, Division of Allergy/Immunology, The Ohio State University Wexner Medical Center, Allergy/Immunology Fellow, Division of Allergy and Immunology, Department of Pediatrics, Nationwide Children's Hospital, Columbus, Ohio

MARIA CASTILLO, MD
Driscoll Children's Hospital, South Texas, Texas

ALEXA M.A. DOSS, MD
Division of Pediatric Allergy, Immunology, and Pulmonary Medicine, St. Louis Children's Hospital, St Louis, Missouri

SELINA GIERER, DO, FACAAI, FAAAAI
Associate Professor, University of Kansas Medical Center, Kansas City, Kansas

MITCHELL H. GRAYSON, MD
Professor and Chief, Division of Allergy and Immunology, Department of Pediatrics, Nationwide Children's Hospital, The Ohio State University, Investigator, Center for Clinical and Translational Research, Abigail Wexner Research Institute at Nationwide Children's Hospital, Columbus, Ohio

MICHELLE L. HERNANDEZ, MD, FAAAAI
Professor of Pediatrics, Division of Allergy and Immunology, Department of Pediatrics, University of North Carolina School of Medicine, Chapel Hill, North Carolina

MATTHEW J. KESIC, PhD, PA-C
Associate Professor, Campbell University College of Pharmacy & Health Sciences, Physician Assistant Program, Buies Creek, North Carolina

MARISSA LOVE, MD, FACAAI, FAAAAI
Assistant Professor, University of Kansas Medical Center, Kansas City, Kansas

JENNILEE LUEDDERS, MD
Division of Allergy and Immunology, Department of Internal Medicine, College of Medicine, University of Nebraska Medical Center, Omaha, Nebraska

CAROLINE L. MORTELLITI, MS
Boston Children's Hospital, Boston, Massachusetts

SYED SHAHZAD MUSTAFA, MD
Clinical Associate Professor of Medicine, Rochester Regional Health, University of Rochester School of Medicine and Dentistry, Rochester, New York

ANIL NANDA, MD
Allergist/Immunologist, Division of Allergy and Immunology, Asthma and Allergy Center, Lewisville and Flower Mound, Texas, Clinical Associate Professor of Medicine, Division of Allergy and Immunology, The University of Texas Southwestern Medical Center, Dallas, Texas

WANDA PHIPATANAKUL, MD, MS
Boston Children's Hospital, Attending Physician, Division of Immunology, Director, Research Center, Division of Immunology, Professor of Pediatrics, Harvard Medical School, Boston, Massachusetts

BROOKE I. POLK, MD
Assistant Professor of Pediatrics, Division of Allergy and Pulmonary Medicine, Washington University in Saint Louis School of Medicine, St Louis, Missouri

JILL A. POOLE, MD
Professor, Division of Allergy and Immunology, Department of Internal Medicine, College of Medicine, University of Nebraska Medical Center, Omaha, Nebraska

JENNY RESILIAC, BS
Biomedical Sciences Graduate Program, The Ohio State University College of Medicine, Center for Translational and Clinical Research, Abigail Wexner Research Institute at Nationwide Children's Hospital, Columbus, Ohio

ANDREW RORIE, MD
Assistant Professor, Department of Medicine, Division of Allergy and Immunology, University of Nebraska Medical Center, Omaha, Nebraska

MEHR ZAHRA SHAH, MD
Resident in Pediatrics, Washington University in Saint Louis School of Medicine, St Louis, Missouri

JEFFREY R. STOKES, MD
Division of Pediatric Allergy, Immunology, and Pulmonary Medicine, St. Louis Children's Hospital, St Louis, Missouri

CAROLINA ZILLI VIEIRA, PhD, DDS
Exposure Epidemiology and Risk Program, Harvard TH Chan School of Public Health, Boston, Massachusetts, USA

CONTENTS

Ozone (O_3) is a ubiquitous outdoor air pollutant, which may be derived from various primary pollutants such as nitrates, hydrocarbons, and volatile organ compounds through ultraviolet radiation exposure, and has been shown to negatively impact respiratory health. O_3 is the most common noninfectious environmental cause of asthma exacerbations among children and adults. Its effects on pediatric respiratory health could be due to multiple physiologic factors that may contribute to enhanced O_3 exposure seen in children compared with adults, including differences in lung surface area per unit of body weight and ventilation rates. O_3 can reach the distal regions of human lungs due to its low water solubility, resulting in either injury or activation of airway epithelial cells and macrophages. Multiple epidemiologic studies have highlighted a link between exposure to air pollution and the development of asthma. This review article specifically focuses on examining the impact of early life O_3 exposure on lung development, lung function, and the risk of developing atopic diseases including asthma, allergic rhinitis, and atopic dermatitis among children.

The pathophysiology of asthma development is heterogenous. Although complex interactions between factors are present in any one individual, early life viral infections have been shown to play a major role through induction of epithelial damage as well as various innate and adaptive immune responses. The cytokine profile that results from epithelial damage leads to Th2 skewing of the adaptive immune response. Most asthma exacerbations in children and up to half of adults are related to viral infections that also induce epithelial damage and an acute predominately Th2 inflammatory response, leading to acute symptoms and chronic airway remodeling.

Wheezing is common in childhood, although only a small percentage of these children develop asthma. The child's wheezing phenotype and asthma predictive indices help predict the likelihood of a future asthma diagnosis. Viral infections are common in childhood with most wheezing episodes due to respiratory syncytial virus and rhinovirus. Many treatment options exist for wheezing children including both those who wheeze persistently and those who wheeze intermittently due to viral infections.

> The school is a microenvironment well-known to host many indoor aller-
> gens and pollutants, with a strong association between school allergen
> exposure and childhood asthma morbidity. Despite advances in therapies,
> asthma continues to be one of the most common chronic conditions
> among children, associated with significant morbidity, health care utiliza-
> tion, and productivity loss. Asthma prevalence is also disproportionately
> high among children in minority communities. This review will focus on
> environmental exposures associated with asthma morbidity (cockroach,
> mouse, cat and dog, dust mite, fungus, air pollution). This review will
> also discuss recent school-based interventions to improve allergy
> morbidity among school-aged children. Understanding the multifaceted
> environmental factors which may contribute to asthma pathogenesis is
> necessary to help guide potential school-based interventions.

> Eosinophilic esophagitis (EoE) is a chronic, non-IgE immune-mediated re-
> action characterized by eosinophilic infiltration leading to esophageal
> dysfunction, inflammation, and potential for fibrotic remodeling. Although
> food allergens are generally considered the leading trigger for EoE,
> emerging evidence suggests that modifiable environmental factors may
> also play a role in the pathogenesis of EoE. This article discusses the latest
> data regarding the role of the exposome, microbiome, and environmental
> allergens on the development and ongoing inflammation of EoE, focusing
> on the last 10 years of relevant studies.

> There is clear evidence that climate change is occurring as there has been
> an acceleration of global temperatures since the mid-nineteenth century
> along with rising atmospheric carbon dioxide levels. It has been proposed
> that one of the most significant consequences of climate change on hu-
> man health could be the impact on aeroallergens. Evidence from around
> globe has pointed to longer and more abundant pollen season associated
> with global warming. Additional studies have also suggested increased
> pollen allergenicity due to air pollution.

> Electronic nicotine delivery systems (ENDS) were introduced in 2006, of-
> fering alternatives to combustible cigarettes. There is significant contro-
> versy regarding their sale and regulation, particularly with youth and
> high-risk patient populations. They were deemed a "major public health
> concern" by the United States (US) Surgeon General in 2016 . Already
> associated with health consequences, recently e-cig or vaping product
> use-associated lung injury (EVALI) has exposed their potential to cause

life-threatening complications. This publication aims to educate readers on the the immediate and long-term health consequences of ENDS, so they may provide patient counseling on utilization focusing on the asthmatic population.

Air Pollution Effects in Allergies and Asthma

Anil Nanda, Syed Shahzad Mustafa, Maria Castillo, and Jonathan A. Bernstein

Outdoor air pollution is associated with exacerbations of allergic diseases, including asthma, allergic rhinitis, and other atopic conditions. The increased allergic disease prevalence has been linked to urbanization, industrialization, and economic growth globally. Air pollutants are well-known to disrupt the epithelium leading to specific diseases in any organ system that has epithelial linings. This review provides an overview of the health effects of air pollution on allergic disorders and specifically addresses how it may impact the epithelial barrier in the upper and lower respiratory tracts to facilitate the health effects associated with these exposures.

Influence of Rural Environmental Factors in Asthma

Jennilee Luedders and Jill A. Poole

Purpose: The objective of this article is to review recent literature on the implications of agricultural factors including pesticides, animal/livestock production facilities, agricultural dust, endotoxin, biomass/crop burning, and nutritional factors with respiratory health. Methods: PubMed, Embase, and CINAHL literature searches for the years 2016 to 2021 were conducted with librarian assistance. Results: Several studies suggest increased risk for asthma or wheeze with certain rural exposures, particularly for pesticides, livestock production facilities, agricultural dust, and biomass and crop burning. Conclusion: A complex network of environmental factors exists, which may have detrimental effects on the respiratory health of rural residents.

IMMUNOLOGY AND ALLERGY CLINICS OF NORTH AMERICA

SERIES OF RELATED INTEREST

Medical Clinics
https://www.medical.theclinics.com/

THE CLINICS ARE AVAILABLE ONLINE!
Access your subscription at:
www.theclinics.com

Preface

The Environment: Critical Cornerstone of Allergic Diseases

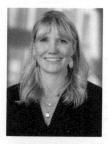

Jill A. Poole, MD
Editor

The environment in which we live represents a fundamental and critical component that drives the development and severity of allergic diseases. Environmental factor patterns are fluid with important shifts observed in the past decades that not only require our recognition but also should transform our approach to allergic diseases. Increased global temperature, carbon dioxide, ozone, and various air pollutants contribute to climate change. One of the most significant consequences of climate change could be its impact on aeroallergens, leading to enhanced pollen burden, longer pollen seasons, and potentially, enhanced allergenicity. These changes also contribute to extreme weather events, including hurricanes, wildfires, drought, and dust storms, that strongly influence allergic disease exacerbations. Vulnerable populations include children, elderly, those with disabilities, and the impoverished, among other groups. Air pollution and particulate matter, including metals and gaseous pollutants (ie, ozone, nitrogen dioxide, sulfur dioxide, and traffic-related air pollution), increase free radicals and reduce antioxidants, leading to airway inflammation, inflammatory cytokine release, oxidative stress, and cellular damage, all associated with new onset and exacerbation of allergic diseases. Dysregulation of the airway epithelial barrier of the upper and lower respiratory tract is an important underlying mechanism explaining air pollutant-associated respiratory disease. Ozone, derived from various primary pollutants, such as nitrates, hydrocarbons, and volatile organic compounds through UV radiation exposure, is the most common noninfectious environmental cause of asthma exacerbations among children and adults. Early life ozone exposure impacts lung development, lung function, and the risk of developing atopic diseases, including asthma, allergic rhinitis, and atopic dermatitis among children. A complex network of environmental factors, including exposure to pesticides, animal production facilities, agricultural dusts, endotoxin, and biomass and crop burning, also have detrimental respiratory health effects. Selective airborne viruses (eg, respiratory syncytial virus, rhinovirus, and parainfluenza virus 1

Immunol Allergy Clin N Am 42 (2022) ix–x
https://doi.org/10.1016/j.iac.2022.06.003
0889-8561/22/© 2022 Published by Elsevier Inc.

and 3) resulting in infections, particularly early in life, impact the development and severity of asthma for years to come. The mechanisms by which respiratory infections are associated with asthma inception are complex and vary by atopic conditions. Viral-induced epithelial damage, however, is a common initial step in the pathway toward asthma development. The school environment hosts many indoor allergens and pollutants (ie, cockroach, mouse, cat, dog, dust mite, mold, air pollutants) with strong associations demonstrated between school allergen exposure and childhood disease. Understanding school-based interventions to improve allergic diseases is necessary. Eosinophilic esophagitis, a disease predominately driven by food allergens, is also increasingly recognized to be influenced by environmental factors with prenatal and early life exposures, genetics, exposomes, and aeroallergens contributing to the multifactorial pathogenesis of the disease. In the hopes of eliminating tobacco smoke exposures, electronic nicotidine delivery systems or vaping use has been increasing since its introduction in 2006, including youth populations. Whereas the outbreak of e-cigarette or vaping product use associated lung injury exposed a threat of potential life-threatening complications from use, and evidence suggests potential airway epithelial cell dysregulation, data are still needed to understand the long-term consequences of these electronic nicotine delivery systems.

In conclusion, raising awareness of the multitude of environmental factors that strongly influence allergic diseases and understanding the need for mitigation strategies as outlined in this issue of *Immunology and Allergy Clinics of North America* should be of great interest among clinicians, researchers, and patients. I am extremely grateful to all the authors who contributed their invaluable expertise and time to produce this high-quality issue. I would like to thank Dr Lanny Rosenwasser, who created the opportunity to publish this issue on "Environmental Issue and Allergy," and Jessica Cañaberal, for her outstanding editorial support.

Jill A. Poole, MD
Allergy and Immunology Division
Department of Internal Medicine
University of Nebraska Medical Center
985990 Nebraska Medical Center
Omaha, NE 68198-5990, USA

E-mail address:
japoole@unmc.edu

Ozone in the Development of Pediatric Asthma and Atopic Disease

Claire E. Atkinson, MD[a,1], Matthew J. Kesic, PhD, PA-C[b,1,2], Michelle L. Hernandez, MD[a,*]

KEYWORDS

- Asthma • Ozone • Children • Lung function • Allergic rhinitis • Atopic dermatitis

KEY POINTS

- Preclinical models show that O_3 exposure during lung development causes morphologic and structural changes.
- Ozone (O_3) exposures over the short term are associated with reduced lung function in both children and adults, independent of asthma status.
- The effects of O_3 exposure during the prenatal and infancy periods on long-term lung growth need to be further evaluated.
- Ozone exposure during early life increases the risk of developing asthma, allergic rhinitis, and atopic dermatitis; effects on food allergy and eosinophilic esophagitis are unknown.

INTRODUCTION

Air pollution is an umbrella term used to describe the presence of substances in the atmosphere that are harmful to humans and other living organisms. These pollutants are also influenced by weather patterns. The most common air pollutants are ground-level ozone (O_3) and particulate matter (PM). Anthropogenic activities such as burning of fossil fuels, deforestation, land use, livestock production, fertilization, and industrial processes have increased greenhouse gas (GHG) emissions and ground-level O_3 production.[1] The increase in air pollution not only has had an impact on climate change but also on public and individual health.[2]

[a] Division of Allergy & Immunology, Department of Pediatrics, University of North Carolina School of Medicine, Chapel Hill, NC, USA; [b] Campbell University College of Pharmacy & Health Sciences, Physician Assistant Program, Buies Creek, NC, USA
[1] The authors contributed equally to this work.
[2] Present address: Tracey F. Smith Hall of Nursing & Health Sciences, Room 216H, 143 Main Street, Buies Creek, NC 27506.
* Corresponding author. 5008C Mary Ellen Jones Building, 116 Manning Drive, CB #7231, Chapel Hill, NC 27599-7231.
E-mail address: michelle_hernandez@med.unc.edu

Immunol Allergy Clin N Am 42 (2022) 701–713
https://doi.org/10.1016/j.iac.2022.06.001
0889-8561/22/© 2022 Elsevier Inc. All rights reserved.
immunology.theclinics.com

It is estimated that roughly 40% of Americans—more than 135 million people—are living in areas that have unhealthy levels of O_3 or particle pollution.[3] While O_3 present in the stratosphere is protective, it is harmful when present in high concentrations at ground level.[4] When inhaled, O_3 has deleterious effects on the respiratory and cardio-vascular systems.[5] Individuals with underlying lung pathology such as asthma are at a higher risk for symptom severity and exacerbations.[2] The pediatric population is also at higher risk for lung pathologies due to several factors, most notably the anatomic differences of the airway and lungs during early development.

Asthma is one of the most common causes of morbidity and hospitalizations in childhood.[6] Studies have shown evidence that asthma is a complex and dynamic disease influenced by many environmental and genetic factors.[7] Asthma exacerbations are a major cause of disease morbidity and are responsible for significantly higher health care costs.[8] Patients that require emergency department (ED) visits/hospitalizations for an exacerbation are at a significantly higher risk for future exacerbations and hospitalizations.[9] Although the exact mechanism(s) for the development of early childhood asthma have yet to be elucidated, evidence has shown that air pollution plays a significant role in both the development and exacerbation of asthma.

It is well established that O_3 exposure increases the risk of asthma exacerbations among children [recently reviewed by[10]]. As children are typically active outside, especially during the warm seasons when O_3 levels are highest, this poses a greater risk of exposure to this air pollutant and subsequent adverse health effects. Because children's respiratory systems are continuously growing and developing through their early 20s,[11] O_3 exposure has the potential to disrupt this normal developmental process through its ability to alter structural elements of conducting airways through long-term oxidative stress of the airways.[12] These exposures may impact future lung function, airway remodeling, and airway hyperreactivity. This review focuses on how O_3 exposure(s) during early life impact lung development, lung function, and the future risk of pediatric asthma and atopic disease.

OZONE PRODUCTION

Ozone is an invisible gas that can be found in different locations in the atmosphere and can serve as both beneficial and hazardous to our health depending on whereby it is found. O_3 that is found in the upper atmosphere, or stratospheric O_3, is classified as "good O_3" and serves as protection from the sun's ultraviolet (UV) radiation. The O_3 that is located at ground-level, or tropospheric, is classified as "bad O_3."[4] Ground-level O_3 is created by chemical reactions that occur when oxides of nitrogen (NOx) and volatile organic compounds (VOC) react in the presence of sunlight. Emissions from industrial facilities, farms, factories, power plants, and motor vehicle exhaust are some of the major sources of NOx and VOC.[4,13] Ground-level O_3 is most likely to reach dangerous and unhealthy levels on hot sunny days. O_3 levels can fluctuate due to altering weather patterns.[1] O_3 can reach the distal aspects of the human airways due to its low water solubility. Once in the airway, it has been shown to increase inflammation, increase susceptibility to viral infections, and promote remodeling of the airway epithelium.[14,15]

SUSCEPTIBILITY OF THE DEVELOPING LUNG TO AIR POLLUTION

Exposure to early life risk factors, including environmental pollutants, plays a critical role in the development and severity of asthma.[6,7] A child's developing respiratory system is extremely vulnerable to O_3 for several reasons. Early in life, the respiratory system is rapidly growing. At the time of birth, the human lung has about 24 million alveoli.[16] This represents a fraction of the remaining alveoli that will develop into a fully functioning respiratory system comprising roughly 257 million alveoli. It is estimated that nearly 80% of the alveoli will develop postnatally and continue to expand throughout adolescence.[17] Additionally, children have a larger lung surface area per kilogram body weight ratio and increased resting respiratory rate compared with adults, corresponding to increased overall exposure.[18] Finally, the smaller caliber of children's airways contributes to their increased susceptibility to air pollution's effects.[18]

The processes of lung growth and development along with how the tissue responds to insults are highly interlinked during early life when there are phases of rapid differentiation and growth.[19] It has been hypothesized that early exposures to risk factors can alter the respiratory system, including lung development and growth, immune development and function, and inflammatory responses to oxidative stress and infections. This process is referred to as "early life programming."[20] The timing and nature of these events result in differing degrees of impaired maximal lung functional capacity in early adulthood, and potentially impact future long-term respiratory morbidities such as chronic asthma or chronic obstructive airway disease (COPD).

OZONE EFFECTS ON LUNG DEVELOPMENT IN PRECLINICAL STUDIES

Ozone exposure has been linked with reductions in children's lung function,[21] but the exact pathophysiology has yet to be illustrated. Most studies that have investigated this were performed in animal models such as rodents. These studies are discussed in more detail elsewhere,[22] but the results from the rodent studies showed mixed and minimal morphologic changes in the airways and lungs.[23–25] This is most likely due to the differences between the development of the human and animal lung. The use of nonhuman primates showed more robust data on O_3 effects due to their similarities with human airway structure and postnatal lung developmental processes.

Neurogenic mechanisms are implicated in airway remodeling from O_3 exposure. A large portion of lung development occurs postnatally.[26,27] These processes include intricate nerve connections/innervations along with the expression of neurotransmitters in the developing respiratory tract.[28,29] Airway nerves/innervation plays a crucial role in maintaining lung function and homeostasis. This is dependent on the specific projection of axons to their targets during lung development.[30] Evidence suggested that the postnatal developmental period is critical for proper lung development and function. During this time the tissue is highly susceptibility to exposures to mild irritants or toxicants that can markedly modify lung development.[25,31,32] Studies using newborn rats demonstrated that early O_3 exposure (postnatal days 2–6) but not late exposure (days 19–23) increased airway sensory nerves, suggesting a narrow window of neural development and plasticity.[24]

Primate models have shown that exposure to O_3 and allergens during early lung development alters structural components of the conducting airways, including innervation and neurokinin-1 receptor (NK-1R) expression which are linked to the development of asthma.[33] This study showed early O_3 exposure results in persistent effects within the airways which resets the steady state so that NK-1R expression is increased in airways.

Studies using Rhesus macaques demonstrated that O_3 exposure during the first year of life resulted in structural changes in the lung along with a decrease in epithelial nerves in midlevel intrapulmonary airways.[27] Follow-up studies demonstrated that despite abatement of allergen and/or O_3 exposure, adaptive mechanisms were still in place that led to an exaggerated increase in airway nerve density and atypical nerve distribution compared with control animals.[34] This indicated that postnatal exposure to allergen and O_3 leads to the hyperinnervation of the pulmonary epithelium and disrupts processes that are important in the establishment of normal airway innervation and may lead to the initiation and persistence of airways disease in children.[34] Studies by Fanucchi and colleagues also used nonhuman primates to study how O_3 alters distal airway development. Using cyclic exposures, it was shown that episodic exposure to O_3 during infancy significantly alters airway morphology and structure. Most notably it was shown that O_3-exposed animals had 4 fewer nonalveolarized airway generations, altered smooth muscle bundle orientation within the terminal and respiratory bronchioles, and hyperplastic bronchiolar epithelium.[35] Taken together, O_3 exposure negatively impacts the developing distal airway morphology resulting in narrower and shorter terminal bronchioles with altered smooth muscle bundles. Normal morphology and structure are critical for proper lung function. It is known that the total amount of smooth muscle is increased in asthma.[36,37] It has also been shown that cell hyperplasia and hypertrophy are present in mild-to-moderate asthma, and even more so in severe asthmatics.[38] One may speculate that these cellular changes are secondary effects brought about by an already ongoing change in the lung microenvironment and immune modulation.

OZONE EFFECTS ON IMMUNE DEVELOPMENT AND FUNCTION

Airway remodeling in asthma is understood to be a response to chronic inflammation. This inflammatory assault requires continuous tissue repair and remodeling, thus a major factor in the development of asthma. Modulation/alteration of the immune cells and response including T helper cells (Th), eosinophils, neutrophils, and mast cells all play a role in the microenvironment of the lung and airway that when under inflammatory conditions result in airway remodeling.

Ozone has been shown to "prime" epithelial inflammatory responses and provokes airway hyperreactivity.[22] Inhaled O_3 does not enter cells but reacts with components of the airway lining fluid to generate other reactive oxygen species (ROS) to enhance local oxidative stress, inflammation, and epithelial cell injury.[39] In response to O_3 exposure, epithelial cells produce proinflammatory mediators, including IL-8, IL-6, prostaglandin E_2 (PGE_2), and leukotriene C_4 (LTC_4), that recruit inflammatory cells [reviewed by [12]]. This damaged epithelial cell-airway lining fluid interface also releases damage-associated molecular patterns (DAMPs), such as heat shock proteins, oxidized lipids, fibrinogen, and low-molecular-weight hyaluronic acid that can then trigger an inflammatory response in airway macrophages. Mouse models have shown that O_3 exposure causes epithelial cell damage and death along with inducing several proinflammatory cytokines including IL-17/IL-22[40] that is mediated by TLR2/TLR4 pathways. Inflammation triggered by O_3 is linked with the development of airway hyperreactivity[41–43] in preclinical models.

OZONE IMPACTS ON LUNG FUNCTION IN CHILDREN

Controlled human exposure studies have consistently observed O_3-associated decrements in lung function and neutrophilic inflammation. O_3-induced, pain-related symptoms may inhibit maximal inspiration due to the stimulation of airway C-fibers, leading to reduced lung function measures[44] that are not necessarily linked to airway inflammatory responses.[44–46] Later in discussion, we review the effects of short-term and long-term ambient O_3 exposures on children's lung function.

IMPACT OF SHORT-TERM EXPOSURES ON LUNG FUNCTION

Multiple studies have evaluated the effects of shorter-term O_3 exposure on lung function in children. A panel study of 97 children ages 10 to 11 years old living in Athens and 89 children living in Thessaloniki followed participants throughout a school year to assess the effects of O_3 exposure on respiratory outcomes, comparing the Forced Vital Capacity (FVC) and Forced Expiratory Volume in 1 Second (FEV_1) values in the fall to values in the spring–summer period.[47] Baseline asthma prevalence among these children ranged from 7% in Athens to 15% in Thessaloniki. Compared with the first spirometry value in the fall, this study found significant decreases, around 5%, in FVC and FEV_1 during the spring–summer period, which was associated with higher O_3 concentrations.[47] In addition, a growth deficit of 0.008% for FVC (~20 mL) was noted over the 6- to 8-month observation period. Additionally, a study of 10,251 healthy White children aged 8 to 12 years in several US and Canadian communities found an almost 3% decrease in FVC and FEV_1 associated with a 37 ug/m^3 increase in O_3 concentrations over the prior year[48]; this effect was seen in both children with and without asthma.

In 2 Austrian studies, 2153 children aged 6 to 9 years had their lung function growth assessed over approximately three 6-month periods classified according to high versus low O_3 concentrations.[49] An asthma diagnosis at the start of the study ranged between 1.2% (Heidenreichstein/Austria) and 12.8% (Amstetten/Austria), and aeroallergen sensitization ranged from 6.8% (Wiesmath/Austria, Ganserndorf/Austria) to 28.8% (Ehingen/Germany). During the summer months, children who had semiannual mean O_3 exposures between 46 and 54 parts per billion (ppb) had a growth deficit of 18.5 mL in FEV_1 and 19.2 mL in FVC compared with children with lower exposures between 22 and 30 ppb. However, over the 3.5-year study period, there was no evident lung function growth deficit; this finding was attributed to the rebound growth that occurred during the winter periods, which compensated for the growth deficits noted during the summer periods.[49]

The impact of O_3 on lung function among children with asthma is also evident in both high and low ambient O_3 environments. One-hundred fifty-eight children with asthma from Mexico City, whereby the mean 1-h maximum O_3 level was 102 ppb (SD 47 ppb) participated in a double-blinded randomized trial to evaluate whether antioxidant vitamin supplementation would attenuate the effects of ambient air pollution.[50] Among children in the placebo group, elevated O_3 concentrations the day before spirometry were significantly associated with reduced forced expiratory flow ($FEF_{25-75\%}$) of 13.32 mL/s and reduced FEV_1 of 4.59 mL for every 10 ppb increase in O_3; no association between O_3 and lung function was observed in the supplement group.[50]

These transient reductions in lung function are also evident with lower O_3 exposures in children with underlying airway disease. The Childhood Asthma Management Program (CAMP) enrolled children ages 5 to 12 years from 8 North American cities who had baseline elevated airway reactivity (by methacholine challenge) at study entry. Increased 4-month averages of ambient O_3 were associated with reduced postbronchodilator FEV_1/FVC.[51] Similarly, African American adolescents with persistent asthma had reduced lung function, despite the use of asthma controller medications, with low level increases of ambient air O_3 concentrations (below the 70 ppb National Ambient Air Quality Standard).[52] Specifically, the strongest effect in the reduction of lung function measurements was observed for O_3 concentrations in the 24-h period preceding clinic visits, whereby %predicted FVC was 2.7 points lower.[52] Similar to the transient decrements in lung function seen with controlled low-dose O_3 exposure studies among adults,[53,54] short-term higher concentrations of O_3 are also associated with reduced lung function in children, with or without asthma.

IMPACT OF EARLY-LIFE EXPOSURES ON LUNG FUNCTION

Although studies have shown that short-term O_3 exposure is associated with reduced lung function, data surrounding the relationship between long-term O_3 exposure and lung function over years are inconclusive.[11] For example, a prospective study of 1759 10-year-old children from southern California assessed the long-term effects of air pollution on children's respiratory health. There was no significant evidence that O_3 was associated with any measure of reduced lung function over an 8-year period.[55]

The lack of O_3 effect seen in some studies could be secondary to the timing of exposure during a child's lung development. To identify the effects of O_3 exposure during the early life period, a cross-sectional school-based survey of 1016 Taiwanese children aged 6 to 15 years without a history of asthma investigated the impact of lifetime residential exposure to intermediate levels of air pollution on spirometry.[56] Exposure to air pollution was assessed during the first year of life, age 2 to 6 years and lifetime; the lifetime annual average exposure was determined based on the residential history data of the participants and the average air pollution value in each township. Although each 1-ppb increase in O_3 was related to a 0.95% decrease in FEV_1 and 0.93% decrease in FVC when accounting for lifetime annual average exposures to O_3, the effects of O_3 became less significant after 2-pollutant adjustment for PM_{10}.[56] Additionally, a prospective birth cohort of 304 healthy term-born infants assessed the adverse effects of air pollution levels before and after birth on lung function at age 6.[57] Exposure assessment of NO_2, O_3, PM_{10} occurred during pregnancy and during the first and sixth years of life. There were 232 children who remained in the study at the 6-year follow-up visit whereby spirometry was performed. While NO_2 exposure during pregnancy and first year of life was associated with decreased FEV_1, there were no significant associations observed for either O_3 or PM_{10}.[57]

In contrast, a large prospective 2-year follow-up study of more than 1300 young children in the Korean Children's Health and Environmental Research (CHEER) cohort (mean age 6.83 ± 0.52 years at enrollment) found that exposure to elevated levels of O_3 within the past 5 years was associated with slight but significant reductions in % predicted FEV_1 and $FEF_{25-75\%}$ that was further amplified by a prior diagnosis of bronchiolitis.[58] Thus, most studies suggest that early life O_3 exposure does not by itself have long-lasting effects on lung growth and function among children. However, the CHEER cohort highlights that air pollutant exposure in the context of prior lung damage may impair future lung function. The long-term effects of O_3 on the lung function of young children with recurrent wheezing who go on to develop future asthma are unclear.

IMPACT OF PRENATAL AND EARLY LIFE EXPOSURES ON ASTHMA DEVELOPMENT

There has been growing interest surrounding the impact of air pollutant exposure during birth and early life on the development of asthma. Although multiple epidemiologic studies throughout the world have linked O_3 exposure with asthma exacerbation and increased respiratory symptoms among children and adults,[10] limited studies to date have specifically examined the effect of in utero or early life O_3 exposure on the risk of subsequent asthma development. Herein we review the studies focused on asthma development from North America and Asia.

A large Canadian birth cohort study followed 65,254 children from birth until age 10 years using linked administrative health databases to evaluate the association between in utero exposure to air pollution and childhood asthma.[59,60] This study found that higher in utero exposure to traffic-related air pollution was associated with increased asthma risk in preschool age children (diagnosed through age 5 years), but that O_3 exposure itself was associated with reduced risk in this age group; this finding was attributed to the negative correlation of O_3 levels with traffic-related air pollutants.[59,60] However, higher in utero O_3 exposure was associated with increased of asthma development among school-aged children (diagnosed after age 6) from this same cohort.[60] Another birth cohort study from Canada followed 1286 children from birth through age 17 to identify risk of air pollution on asthma and atopic disease.[61] In a single-pollutant model, O_3 exposure at birth was not associated with asthma, allergic rhinitis, or eczema; however, in a multi-pollutant model that adjusted for NO_2, $PM_{2.5}$ and Normalized Difference Vegetation Index (NDVI), there was a 1.2-fold higher risk of asthma per interquartile range (IQR) increase in O_3 exposure at birth. The findings were more robust when accounting for oxidant pollutants (both O_3 and NO_2) whereby for each IQR increase in oxidant pollutant exposure at birth, there was a 17% increase in the risk of developing asthma and 8% increase in risk of allergic rhinitis.[61] Similarly, another population-based birth cohort study of Canadian children born in Québec between 1996 and 2011 assessed the association between outdoor air pollutant exposures at birth and the onset of childhood asthma.[62] Asthma onset in children was associated with birth residential exposure to $PM_{2.5}$, O_3, and NO_2, with a Hazard Ratio (HR) of 1.06 (1.05–1.07) per interquartile range increase of O_3 levels.[62]

Among Latino children and young adults living the in the mainland United States and Puerto Rico in urban areas, the Genes-environments & Admixture in Latino Americans (GALA II) study found that for every 5 ppb increase in average O_3 exposure during the first year of life, the odds for having asthma without allergic sensitization increased by 32%.[63] Additionally, children with asthma without allergic sensitization were more likely to be exposed to higher levels of O_3 during the first year of life compared with children with atopic asthma, suggesting that mechanisms independent of atopy [such as airway neutrophilia seen in nonatopic children[64]] may account for promoting asthma development.

Early life cohort studies in Asia have found similarities between early life O_3 exposure and asthma development. The Prenatal Environments and Offspring Health (PEOH cohort) that followed 3725 mother–child dyads from Guangzhou, China, recently found that elevated O_3 exposure increased the risk of preschool wheezing.[65] Additionally, the risk of preschool wheezing was further amplified if maternal O_3 exposure occurred during warm weather months (when ambient O_3 exposures are elevated). A population-based cohort study of more than 30,000 children in China aged 2 to 14 years observed a significant relationship between doctor-diagnosed asthma and increases in O_3 exposure average for the preceding 3 years before assessment.[66] This positive association was seen in both normal weight (Odds Ratio, OR 1.25 (1.12, 1.40) and overweight/obese children (OR 1.41 (1.22, 1.63). Additionally, elementary-school children from the CHEER cohort in Korea that had exposure to elevated levels of O_3 within the past 5 years and prior episodes of bronchiolitis had a significantly higher prevalence of current asthma and greater nonspecific airway reactivity assessed by methacholine challenge.[58]

In summary, the available epidemiologic evidence is stronger in support of early life O_3 exposure increasing the risk of future asthma. Although O_3 exposure may not have long-lasting effects on lung function growth, by spirometry, preclinical studies support that O_3 alters airway innervation and smooth muscle bundles that would impact nonspecific bronchial reactivity, one of the hallmarks of asthma.

ALLERGIC RHINITIS

Prior studies have reported that the effects of O_3, including bronchial and bronchiolar injury and tissue hypoxia, are associated with higher risk of diseases such as allergic rhinitis. The evidence surrounding allergic rhinitis development with O_3 exposure is mixed. A longitudinal birth cohort study of 1286 Canadian children, aged 5 to 9 years, who were followed for an average of 17 years assessed the impact of O_3 exposure in the first 3 years of life whereby O_3 exposures were estimated for the months of May to October (8-h daily maximum) using a temporally adjusted model combining modeled O_3 from the Canadian Hemispheric Regional O_3 and NO_x system operational regional air quality forecast model with ground-based observations from monitors in Canada and the US.[61] Exposure to O_3 at birth was associated with 1.2-fold higher risk of allergic rhinitis when adjusting for NO_2, $PM_{2.5}$, and NDVI in the multi-pollutant model. Similar to what this group reported with increased risk of asthma, increased exposures to total oxidants (NO_2 and O_3) in the first 3 years of life was associated with an increasing the risk of allergic rhinitis development.[61]

A large cross-sectional study in China examined the effects of air pollution on children between the ages of 2 to 17 years old living in Liaoning Province, a highly industrialized region in northeastern China.[67] Four years before the investigation, ambient O_3 exposure was estimated by using a satellite-based random forest model. Long-term exposure to O_3 was significantly associated with higher risk of allergic rhinitis, which was more pronounced in children aged 7 to 17 years.[67]

Additionally, the impact of O_3 exposure on the development of allergic rhinitis was evaluated in school-aged children who reside in industrial areas in Korea, whereby the O_3 concentration was higher[58] using a prospective survey of parental responses to the International Study of Asthma and Allergies in Childhood (ISAAC) questionnaires along with an evaluation for atopic status including total and allergen-specific IgE. During the 2-year study period, there was an increased rate of newly developed sensitization to outdoor allergens in children exposed to the higher levels of O_3, and there was a significant increase in the lifetime prevalence of allergic rhinitis.[58] This could suggest that O_3 exposure may promote the development of sensitization to environmental allergens. Most pediatric studies reviewed showed a positive association between O_3 exposure and allergic rhinitis development.

FOOD ALLERGY AND ATOPIC DERMATITIS

No studies to date have examined the relationship between O_3 exposure and the development of food allergy or eosinophilic esophagitis. Overall, there are limited studies that examine the relationship between O_3 exposure and development of atopic dermatitis in children. A Korean study assessed the association between hospitalization for atopic dermatitis and ambient O_3 levels in children less than 15 years old in the years 2004 to 2005. They found a higher relative risk of childhood atopic dermatitis in Ulsan, a highly industrialized Korean city with higher O_3 concentrations, compared with Seoul, a centrally located in the Korean peninsula with lower O_3 concentrations.[68] A longitudinal birth cohort study of 1286 Canadian children, aged 5 to 9 years, assessed the impact of O_3 exposure during the first 3 years of life. While O_3 exposure at birth was not associated with eczema in single-pollutant models, they found exposures to total oxidants (NO_2 and O_3) in the first 3 years of life showed a similar trend of increasing the risk of eczema in the multi-pollutant model (similar to what was reported with increased risk of comorbid allergic rhinitis and asthma).[61]

SUMMARY

Preclinical studies and more recent epidemiologic studies support that early life exposure to O_3 increases susceptibility to developing chronic airway disease including asthma and allergic rhinitis (**Fig. 1**). Once asthma is established, elevated O_3 levels are well known to cause asthma exacerbations in both children and adults. In addition

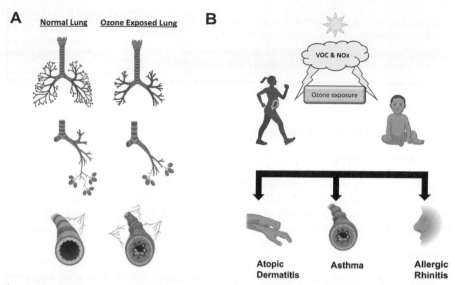

Fig. 1. Ozone exposure and the development of asthma and atopic disease. (*A*). Ozone exposure during lung development causes morphologic and structural changes: decreases bronchial branching and alveoli number, alterations in smooth muscle bundle orientation, and hyperinnervation of pulmonary epithelium. (*B*). Ozone exposure during early life increases the risk of developing asthma, allergic rhinitis, and atopic dermatitis. (Created with BioRender.com.)

to promoting neutrophil-predominant airway inflammation, O_3 may increase the risk of allergic sensitization[58] and enhance the response to environmental allergens[69] that further perpetuate a prolonged airway inflammatory response. Such chronic inflammation may contribute to airway remodeling seen with chronic respiratory diseases such as asthma and COPD.[12]

The evidence underlying the impact of O_3 on adverse health effects compelled the US Environmental Protection Agency (EPA) to lower the primary and secondary National Ambient Air Quality Standard (NAAQS) for O_3 to 70 ppb in 2015.[70] Primary standards are meant to provide protective for "sensitive" populations who may have increased susceptibility to air pollution, namely children, the elderly, and those with underlying respiratory diseases such as asthma, while secondary standards are meant to provide widespread protection and promote public welfare. Based on our review, much work still needs to be conducted to address the potential effects of prolonged O_3 exposure at levels below the NAAQS on pregnant persons and infants that would impact early life lung development, asthma inception, and the development of other allergic diseases such as atopic dermatitis, food allergy, and eosinophilic esophagitis. These data are needed to develop robust, evidence-based policies that will reduce the overall burden of ambient air pollution for future generations throughout the globe.

CLINICS CARE POINTS

- O_3 is the most common noninfectious environmental cause of asthma exacerbations: it is imperative to minimize O_3 exposure among children and adults with underlying respiratory disease.

- Ozone exposure of pregnant persons and young children should be minimized to reduce the risk of developing asthma, allergic rhinitis, and atopic dermatitis.
- Clinical studies are needed to evaluate any links between O_3 exposure and risk of developing other atopic diseases such as food allergy and eosinophilic esophagitis.

CONFLICTS OF INTEREST

The authors have nothing to disclose.

ACKNOWLEDGEMENTS

Research reported in this publication was supported by the National Institutes of Health under award numbers NHLBI R01HL135235 and NCATS UL1TR002489. The content is solely the responsibility of the authors and does not necessarily represent the official views of the NIH.

REFERENCES

1. Pacheco SE, Guidos-Fogelbach G, Annesi-Maesano I, et al. American Academy of Allergy A, Immunology Environmental E, Respiratory Health C. Climate change and global issues in allergy and immunology. J Allergy Clin Immunol 2021;148: 1366–77.
2. Pfeffer PE, Mudway IS, Grigg J. Air Pollution and Asthma: Mechanisms of Harm and Considerations for Clinical Interventions. Chest 2021;159:1346–55.
3. Association AL. State of the air: 2021. Chicago, IL: Association AL; 2021. p. 11.
4. EPA U. Ground Level Ozone. 2022 2022. Available at: https://www.epa.gov/ground-level-ozone-pollution/ground-level-ozone-basics#wwh. Accessed March 2, 2022.
5. Bourdrel T, Bind MA, Bejot Y, et al. Cardiovascular effects of air pollution. Arch Cardiovasc Dis 2017;110:634–42.
6. Decrue F, Gorlanova O, Usemann J, et al. Correction to: Lung functional development and asthma trajectories. Semin Immunopathol 2020;42:227.
7. Pavord ID, Beasley R, Agusti A, et al. After asthma: redefining airways diseases. Lancet 2018;391:350–400.
8. Ivanova JI, Bergman R, Birnbaum HG, et al. Effect of asthma exacerbations on health care costs among asthmatic patients with moderate and severe persistent asthma. J Allergy Clin Immunol 2012;129:1229–35.
9. Miller MK, Lee JH, Miller DP, et al. Recent asthma exacerbations: a key predictor of future exacerbations. Respir Med 2007;101:481–9.
10. Li X, Chen Q, Zheng X, et al. Effects of ambient ozone concentrations with different averaging times on asthma exacerbations: A meta-analysis. Sci Total Environ 2019;691:549–61.
11. Garcia E, Rice MB, Gold DR. Air pollution and lung function in children. J Allergy Clin Immunol 2021;148:1–14.
12. Auerbach A, Hernandez ML. The effect of environmental oxidative stress on airway inflammation. Curr Opin Allergy Clin Immunol 2012;12:133–9.
13. Chung KF, Togbe D, Ryffel B. Editorial: Ozone as a Driver of Lung Inflammation and Innate Immunity and as a Model for Lung Disease. Front Immunol 2021; 12:714161.
14. Mumby S, Chung KF, Adcock IM. Transcriptional Effects of Ozone and Impact on Airway Inflammation. Front Immunol 2019;10:1610.

15. Kesic MJ, Meyer M, Bauer R, et al. Exposure to ozone modulates human airway protease/antiprotease balance contributing to increased influenza A infection. PLoS One 2012;7:e35108.
16. Schwartz J. Air pollution and children's health. Pediatrics 2004;113:1037–43.
17. Dietert RR, Etzel RA, Chen D, et al. Workshop to identify critical windows of exposure for children's health: immune and respiratory systems work group summary. Environ Health Perspect 2000;108(Suppl 3):483–90.
18. Landrigan PJ, Kimmel CA, Correa A, et al. Children's health and the environment: public health issues and challenges for risk assessment. Environ Health Perspect 2004;112:257–65.
19. Postma DS, Bush A, van den Berge M. Risk factors and early origins of chronic obstructive pulmonary disease. Lancet 2015;385:899–909.
20. Shaheen S, Barker DJ. Early lung growth and chronic airflow obstruction. Thorax 1994;49:533–6.
21. Romieu I, Samet JM, Smith KR, et al. Outdoor air pollution and acute respiratory infections among children in developing countries. J Occup Environ Med 2002;44:640–9.
22. Auten RL, Foster WM. Biochemical effects of ozone on asthma during postnatal development. Biochim Biophys Acta 2011;1810:1114–9.
23. Shore SA, Abraham JH, Schwartzman IN, et al. Ventilatory responses to ozone are reduced in immature rats. J Appl Physiol (1985) 2000;88:2023–30.
24. Hunter DD, Wu Z, Dey RD. Sensory neural responses to ozone exposure during early postnatal development in rat airways. Am J Respir Cell Mol Biol 2010;43:750–7.
25. Johnston CJ, Holm BA, Finkelstein JN. Differential proinflammatory cytokine responses of the lung to ozone and lipopolysaccharide exposure during postnatal development. Exp Lung Res 2004;30:599–614.
26. Tschanz SA, Burri PH. Postnatal lung development and its impairment by glucocorticoids. Pediatr Pulmonol Suppl 1997;16:247–9.
27. Larson SD, Schelegle ES, Walby WF, et al. Postnatal remodeling of the neural components of the epithelial-mesenchymal trophic unit in the proximal airways of infant rhesus monkeys exposed to ozone and allergen. Toxicol Appl Pharmacol 2004;194:211–20.
28. Sparrow MP, Weichselbaum M, McCray PB. Development of the innervation and airway smooth muscle in human fetal lung. Am J Respir Cell Mol Biol 1999;20:550–60.
29. Sparrow MP, Lamb JP. Ontogeny of airway smooth muscle: structure, innervation, myogenesis and function in the fetal lung. Respir Physiol Neurobiol 2003;137:361–72.
30. Hinck L. The versatile roles of "axon guidance" cues in tissue morphogenesis. Dev Cell 2004;7:783–93.
31. Plopper CG, Fanucchi MV. Do urban environmental pollutants exacerbate childhood lung diseases? Environ Health Perspect 2000;108:A252–3.
32. McMillan SJ, Lloyd CM. Prolonged allergen challenge in mice leads to persistent airway remodelling. Clin Exp Allergy 2004;34:497–507.
33. Murphy SR, Schelegle ES, Edwards PC, et al. Postnatal exposure history and airways: oxidant stress responses in airway explants. Am J Respir Cell Mol Biol 2012;47:815–23.
34. Kajekar R, Pieczarka EM, Smiley-Jewell SM, et al. Early postnatal exposure to allergen and ozone leads to hyperinnervation of the pulmonary epithelium. Respir Physiol Neurobiol 2007;155:55–63.

35. Fanucchi MV, Plopper CG, Evans MJ, et al. Cyclic exposure to ozone alters distal airway development in infant rhesus monkeys. Am J Physiol Lung Cell Mol Physiol 2006;291:L644–50.

36. Jeffery PK. Remodeling and inflammation of bronchi in asthma and chronic obstructive pulmonary disease. Proc Am Thorac Soc 2004;1:176–83.

37. Fixman ED, Stewart A, Martin JG. Basic mechanisms of development of airway structural changes in asthma. Eur Respir J 2007;29:379–89.

38. Benayoun L, Druilhe A, Dombret MC, et al. Airway structural alterations selectively associated with severe asthma. Am J Respir Crit Care Med 2003;167:1360–8.

39. Bromberg PA. Mechanisms of the acute effects of inhaled ozone in humans. Biochim Biophys Acta 2016;1860:2771–81.

40. Michaudel C, Bataille F, Maillet I, et al. Ozone-Induced Aryl Hydrocarbon Receptor Activation Controls Lung Inflammation via Interleukin-22 Modulation. Front Immunol 2020;11:144.

41. Garantziotis S, Li Z, Potts EN, et al. Hyaluronan mediates ozone-induced airway hyperresponsiveness in mice. J Biol Chem 2009;284:11309–17.

42. Garantziotis S, Li Z, Potts EN, et al. TLR4 is necessary for hyaluronan-mediated airway hyperresponsiveness after ozone inhalation. Am J Respir Crit Care Med 2010;181:666–75.

43. Williams AS, Leung SY, Nath P, et al. Role of TLR2, TLR4, and MyD88 in murine ozone-induced airway hyperresponsiveness and neutrophilia. J Appl Physiol (1985) 2007;103:1189–95.

44. Hazucha MJ, Bates DV, Bromberg PA. Mechanism of action of ozone on the human lung. J Appl Physiol (1985) 1989;67:1535–41.

45. Hazucha MJ, Madden M, Pape G, et al. Effects of cyclo-oxygenase inhibition on ozone-induced respiratory inflammation and lung function changes. Eur J Appl Physiol Occup Physiol 1996;73:17–27.

46. Passannante AN, Hazucha MJ, Bromberg PA, et al. Nociceptive mechanisms modulate ozone-induced human lung function decrements. J Appl Physiol (1985) 1998;85:1863–70.

47. Dimakopoulou K, Douros J, Samoli E, et al. Long-term exposure to ozone and children's respiratory health: Results from the RESPOZE study. Environ Res 2020;182:109002.

48. Raizenne M, Neas LM, Damokosh AI, et al. Health effects of acid aerosols on North American children: pulmonary function. Environ Health Perspect 1996;104:506–14.

49. Ihorst G, Frischer T, Horak F, et al. Long- and medium-term ozone effects on lung growth including a broad spectrum of exposure. Eur Respir J 2004;23:292–9.

50. Romieu I, Sienra-Monge JJ, Ramirez-Aguilar M, et al. Antioxidant supplementation and lung functions among children with asthma exposed to high levels of air pollutants. Am J Respir Crit Care Med 2002;166:703–9.

51. Ierodiakonou D, Zanobetti A, Coull BA, et al. Ambient air pollution, lung function, and airway responsiveness in asthmatic children. J Allergy Clin Immunol 2016;137:390–9.

52. Hernandez ML, Dhingra R, Burbank AJ, et al. Low-level ozone has both respiratory and systemic effects in African American adolescents with asthma despite asthma controller therapy. J Allergy Clin Immunol 2018;142:1974–7.e3.

53. Alexis NE, Lay JC, Zhou H, et al. The glutathione-S-transferase mu 1 (GSTM1) null genotype and increased neutrophil response to low-level ozone (0.06 ppm). J Allergy Clin Immunol 2013;131:610–2.

54. Hernandez ML, Ivins S, Chason K, et al. Respiratory Effects of Sedentary Ozone Exposure at the 70-ppb National Ambient Air Quality Standard: A Randomized Clinical Trial. Am J Respir Crit Care Med 2021;203:910–3.
55. Gauderman WJ, Avol E, Gilliland F, et al. The effect of air pollution on lung development from 10 to 18 years of age. N Engl J Med 2004;351:1057–67.
56. Tsui HC, Chen CH, Wu YH, et al. Lifetime exposure to particulate air pollutants is negatively associated with lung function in non-asthmatic children. Environ Pollut 2018;236:953–61.
57. Usemann J, Decrue F, Korten I, et al. Exposure to moderate air pollution and associations with lung function at school-age: A birth cohort study. Environ Int 2019; 126:682–9.
58. Kim BJ, Seo JH, Jung YH, et al. Air pollution interacts with past episodes of bronchiolitis in the development of asthma. Allergy 2013;68:517–23.
59. Clark NA, Demers PA, Karr CJ, et al. Effect of early life exposure to air pollution on development of childhood asthma. Environ Health Perspect 2010;118:284–90.
60. Sbihi H, Tamburic L, Koehoorn M, et al. Perinatal air pollution exposure and development of asthma from birth to age 10 years. Eur Respir J 2016;47:1062–71.
61. To T, Zhu J, Stieb D, et al. Early life exposure to air pollution and incidence of childhood asthma, allergic rhinitis and eczema. Eur Respir J 2020;55:1900913.
62. Tetreault LF, Doucet M, Gamache P, et al. Childhood Exposure to Ambient Air Pollutants and the Onset of Asthma: An Administrative Cohort Study in Quebec. Environ Health Perspect 2016;124:1276–82.
63. Nishimura KK, Iwanaga K, Oh SS, et al. Early-life ozone exposure associated with asthma without sensitization in Latino children. J Allergy Clin Immunol 2016;138: 1703–6.e1.
64. Drews AC, Pizzichini MM, Pizzichini E, et al. Neutrophilic airway inflammation is a main feature of induced sputum in nonatopic asthmatic children. Allergy 2009;64: 1597–601.
65. Zhu S, Chen G, Ye Y, et al. Effect of maternal ozone exposure before and during pregnancy on wheezing risk in offspring: A birth cohort study in Guangzhou, China. Environ Res 2022;212:113426.
66. Dong GH, Qian Z, Liu MM, et al. Obesity enhanced respiratory health effects of ambient air pollution in Chinese children: the Seven Northeastern Cities study. Int J Obes (Lond) 2013;37:94–100.
67. Zhou PE, Qian ZM, McMillin SE, et al. Relationships between Long-Term Ozone Exposure and Allergic Rhinitis and Bronchitic Symptoms in Chinese Children. Toxics 2021;9:221.
68. Lee JT, Cho YS, Son JY. Relationship between ambient ozone concentrations and daily hospital admissions for childhood asthma/atopic dermatitis in two cities of Korea during 2004-2005. Int J Environ Health Res 2010;20:1–11.
69. Peden DB, Setzer RW Jr, Devlin RB. Ozone exposure has both a priming effect on allergen-induced responses and an intrinsic inflammatory action in the nasal airways of perennially allergic asthmatics. Am J Respir Crit Care Med 1995;151: 1336–45.
70. EPA US. Integrated science assessment of ozone and related photochemical oxidants (final report). Washington, DC: U.S. Environmental Protection Agency; 2013.

Immunopathology of Differing Viral Infection in Allergic Asthma Disease

Jenny Resiliac, BS[a,b,1], Christopher D. Brooks, MD[c,d,1], Mitchell H. Grayson, MD[b,d],*

KEYWORDS

• Asthma • Virus • Viral asthma • Allergic asthma • Asthma development

KEY POINTS

• The pathophysiology of asthma is heterogenous and complex with multiple factors that lead to or are correlated with the development of asthma (such as atopic predisposition; in utero pollution exposure; maternal smoking, alcohol use, and vitamin D deficiency; postnatal vitamin D level; intestinal and respiratory microbiome; and early-life viral infections).

• Early life viral infections contribute to the development asthma with the most common viruses being respiratory syncytial virus, rhinovirus, and parainfluenza virus 1 and parainfluenza virus 3. The mechanisms by which respiratory infections are associated with inception of asthma are complex and vary by atopic conditions. However, viral epithelial damage is a common initial step in the pathway toward asthma development.

• Viruses contribute to most pediatric asthma exacerbations and half of adult exacerbations, mostly mediated by similar innate and adaptive responses that contributed to the initial development of asthma.

[a] Biomedical Sciences Graduate Program, The Ohio State University College of Medicine, 1178 Graves Hall, 333 W. 10th Ave, Columbus, OH 43210, USA; [b] Center for Clinical and Translational Research, Abigail Wexner Research Institute at Nationwide Children's Hospital, 700 Children's Drive, Columbus, OH 43205, USA; [c] Department of Otolaryngology, Division of Allergy/Immunology, The Ohio State University Wexner Medical Center, Eye and Ear Institute, 915 Olentangy River Road, Suite 4000, Columbus, OH 43212, USA; [d] Division of Allergy and Immunology, Department of Pediatrics, Nationwide Children's Hospital, The Ohio State University, 700 Children's Drive, Columbus, OH 43205, USA

[1] Cofirst authors who contributed equally.

* Corresponding author. Division of Allergy and Immunology, Department of Pediatrics, Nationwide Children's Hospital, The Ohio State University, 700 Children's Drive, Columbus, OH 43205.

E-mail address: Mitchell.Grayson@Nationwidechildrens.org
Twitter: @MitchMD (M.H.G.)

Immunol Allergy Clin N Am 42 (2022) 715–726
https://doi.org/10.1016/j.iac.2022.05.003
immunology.theclinics.com

INTRODUCTION/HISTORY/DEFINITIONS/BACKGROUND

Asthma is a heterogenous disorder characterized by airway inflammation, airway hyperresponsiveness, and airflow obstruction. Persistent airway inflammation is a characteristic feature and is accompanied by increased airway smooth muscle mass, thickening of the subepithelial lamina reticularis, matrix deposition throughout the airway, increase in microvasculature and neural innervation, as well as mucous cell metaplasia. With exposure to triggers, acute inflammation can occur that leads to an asthma exacerbation with bronchoconstriction and increased mucus production. Triggers that are associated with asthma exacerbations include allergens, aspirin or nonsteroidal anti-inflammatory drugs, hormones, pollution/smoke, and viral infections.

Asthma is a major public health concern with significant mortality, morbidity, and economic burden worldwide. In 2019, 262 million people were affected by asthma, with 461,000 deaths and 21.6 million disability-adjusted life years worldwide.[1] In the United States alone, 7% of children and 8% of adults suffer from asthma. The disease has a disproportionate effect based on socioeconomic status, with asthma being present in up to 11.0% of those living below the federally defined poverty level.[2] In 2013, the economic burden of asthma in the United States was estimated to be more than $81.9 billion related to losses from missed work and school days, asthma-related mortality, and associated medical costs.[3] Understanding the underlying pathophysiology, especially related to disease development as well as triggers that lead to exacerbations, is critical. Viral infections have been associated with development and exacerbation of asthma. In this review, we focus on the mechanisms by which viral infections affect allergic asthma and ongoing work to further delineate the mechanisms through which viral infections affect asthma disease phenotype.

ROLE OF VIRAL INFECTIONS IN ALLERGIC ASTHMA
Viruses and Atopic Development

Respiratory viruses are common during early life development, and they have been implicated in both the development and exacerbation of asthma, depending on the severity of infection during early life. Nearly all children are affected with respiratory syncytial virus (RSV) and rhinovirus (RV) within the first 2 years of life. Additionally, approximately 60% of the children are infected with parainfluenza virus 3 (PIV-3) by the age of 2 years, and the percentage increases to close to 80% by the time they are aged 4 years.[4] Indeed, many children experience an episode of wheezing within the first few years of life with more than 50% of children having had a wheezing episode by 5 to 6 years of age.[5] Perhaps, not surprisingly, RSV, RV, and parainfluenza viruses (PIV-1 and PIV-3) are the most common viruses identified during these wheezing episodes, and they most likely to contribute to the development and exacerbation of asthma, with a positive correlation between severity of infection and risk.[4,6–10] Interestingly, there are differences in asthma development in atopic and nonatopic individuals. RSV infection poses a greater risk of asthma development in individuals who are nonatopic when affected by a severe RSV infection, whereas RV represents a greater risk factor for wheezing in individuals who have preexisting atopic conditions.[11] Other viruses such as enterovirus, bocavirus, coronavirus, metapneumovirus, influenza virus, and adenovirus have also been identified during wheezing episodes and may play a role in the inception and exacerbation of the disease as well.[12] The mechanisms by which respiratory viral infections are linked to the development of allergic diseases or its exacerbations are actively being studied in mouse models and human studies.

One such mouse model that we have used uses the murine parainfluenza virus, Sendai virus (SeV). Mice infected with SeV develop postviral airway hyper-reactivity and mucous cell metaplasia after clearance of the virus, which is akin to the development of "asthma" in humans. The mechanistic pathway we identified depended on the recruitment of a subset of CD49d-expressing neutrophils, which required cysteinyl leukotrienes for survival. The neutrophils drove expression of the high affinity receptor for IgE, FcεRI, on lung conventional dendritic cells (DCs). Simultaneously, the mouse made IgE against SeV while SeV was still being produced. This allowed for the SeV-IgE to be cross-linked on lung conventional DCs. The cross-linking of DC FcεRI-induced production of CC chemokine ligand 28 (CCL28), a chemokine that recruited interleukin (IL)-13 producing lymphocytes to the lung. IL-13 then drove the subsequent development of postviral airway disease.[13] Interestingly, we found that the exposure to a nonviral antigen (in this case ovalbumin) during the antiviral immune response was sufficient to drive IgE and allergic disease against the nonviral antigen. Thus, this mouse model translated a respiratory viral infection into atopy and asthma. Importantly, components of this pathway are present in the human,[14,15] and humans make IgE against viruses such as RSV and RV.[16-20] Whether this pathway does indeed translate a respiratory viral infection to asthma in human infants remains to be fully determined, as does the functional consequence of antiviral IgE. We discuss this further in the section on viral-induced exacerbations.

Other mouse models have focused on the innate immune response. Airway epithelial cells are the first immune cells that stimulate a response during a viral infection.[21] Several murine models have demonstrated that airway epithelial cells produce a variety of cytokines due to the activation of pathogen-associated molecular patterns (PAMPs) and damage-associated molecular patterns (DAMPs) during the viral infection.[22-24] These cytokines can serve to modulate DCs and recruit other innate immune cells into the airways, leading to increased inflammation. Further, IL-13, in a manner akin to what we see in our SeV model, stimulates increased mucous production, airway hyperresponsiveness, and fibrosis.[25] In a murine RSV model, IL-13 production from lymphocytes was shown to depend on the epithelial cell-derived cytokine, thymic stromal lymphopoietin (TSLP).[26-28] TSLP regulates Th2 cytokine profile by upregulating OX40 ligand (OX40 L) on DCs, leading to the recruitment of Th2 lymphocytes.[29] Blockage of TLSP impaired Th2 responses and led to a reduction in serum IgE and airway eosinophils, highlighting its important role in mediating the allergic inflammatory response.[29] In addition to TSLP, airway epithelial cell-produced cytokines that skew the Th2 response are IL-25 and IL-33.[30] IL-25 is a proinflammatory cytokine that can favor Th2 phenotype and activates DCs and type 2 innate lymphoid cells (ILC2s). Simultaneously, IL-33 is produced by epithelial cells, and it activates Th2 cells and ILC2s to stimulate the production of the Th2 signature cytokine response.[31] Viral infection, more specifically RV infection, has been associated with production of IL-25 and IL-33. The increase in these cytokines promotes airway inflammation and remodeling primarily by ILC2s.[32] A study in which naïve human T cells and ILC2s were cultured with the supernatants of RV-infected bronchial epithelial cells demonstrated that RV-induced IL-33 production by epithelial cells drove skewing of naïve Th cells into Th2 cells, as well as increasing IL-5 and IL-13 production by ILC2s; both of these responses depended on IL-33 receptor expression by the Th cells and ILC2s, respectively.[33]

Another recent study investigated the mechanism by which RV infection affects individuals based on their atopic status. Although subjects with asthma or allergic rhinitis had increased symptoms and elevated eosinophilic inflammation with experimental RV upper airway infection compared with healthy controls, this study found no significant differences in viral titer among these 3 groups.[34] This suggests that although the Th2 phenotype may associate with worsening symptoms, it has little impact on viral clearance. Altogether, these studies suggest innate immunity is critical not only for a robust antiviral immune response but also for skewing the cytokine milieu, leading to atopic conditions and the development of allergic diseases such as asthma but that Th2 atopic milieu does not seem to impair viral clearance.

Interferons (IFNs) are a critical component of the antiviral immune response. Type I IFNs (IFNα and IFNβ) have direct antiviral effects and can suppress the Th2 response as well as IgE production.[35] In infants, increased type I IFN in the respiratory mucosa is associated with protection from RSV infection in line with the antiviral properties of this cytokine. Indeed, results from a cohort study of 219 infants followed for 5 years after RSV infection suggest the presence of mucosal IFNs, correlating with protection against severe RSV disease.[36] In this study, IFN levels, particularly type I and type III (IFNλ), were significantly increased in outpatient infants compared with those hospitalized with severe disease, and in those hospitalized with RSV, elevated IFN levels trended to associate with less need for supportive oxygen for prolonged periods of time (OR: 0.35 [0.11–1.07]; $P = .07$) or extended hospital stay (OR: 0.42 [0.16–1.03]; $P = .06$).[36] Importantly, an impaired type I IFN response was found to associate with increased viral replication and a suboptimally regulated Th2 inflammatory response, as well as increased IL-10 levels in therapy-resistant atopic asthmatic children and infants hospitalized with acute lower airway tract infections.[37,38] IFN-β was identified as one of the key cytokines modulating the antiviral immune response and was shown to be deficient in RV-infected cells from patients with asthma.[39] Although less often considered in antiviral immune responses, type II IFN, or IFN-γ, can prevent Th2 skewing, and during RV and RSV infections in infants, IFN-γ and other innate immunity cytokines in nasal wash samples inversely correlated with disease severity.[40]

Altogether, the literature suggests that a deficient IFN response predisposes young children to viral respiratory infections commonly linked with asthma. The immunologic response to viral infection and the epithelial damage in the setting of reduced IFN responses can lead to Th2 skewing, promoting the development of atopy and allergic asthma.

Viruses and Asthma Exacerbation

Viral infections are also among the most common causes of asthma exacerbations, and studies have reported that 67% to 85% of asthma exacerbation episodes in children occur with respiratory viral infections,[41–43] whereas 50% of exacerbations in adults are thought to be due to a respiratory viral infection.[42] Among asthma patients with a viral-induced exacerbation, RV is the most common viral trigger. In fact, when a causative virus could be identified during an exacerbation, that virus was found to be RV in about 65% of the cases.[44–46] RV consists of 3 major clades, RV-A, RV-B, and RV-C, and among these subtypes, RV-A and RV-C have been most associated with asthma exacerbations.[42,47] Further, RV-C seems to drive more severe exacerbations than RV-A.[47,48]

In addition to being important in the development of the atopic milieu, the innate-to-adaptive immune system also plays an important role in viral-induced asthma exacerbations. DAMPs and PAMPs of stressed and damaged epithelial cells from the viral infection lead to cytokine release and increased cellular recruitment of innate and adaptive immune cells. Through the release of proinflammatory cytokines there is increased cellular recruitment of macrophages, eosinophils, and neutrophils to the airways.[49,50] Neutrophils accumulate in the airway and release neutrophil elastase, which further promotes eosinophilic infiltration and type 2 immune responses,[51] as well as increased mucus production.[52] RSV, in particular, can induce leukotriene C4 synthase expression on bronchial epithelial cells, which promotes and influences eosinophilic inflammation.[53] Because cells involved with airway immunity are already primed toward a Th2 phenotype and away from a Th1 phenotype, there is an overall augmented Th2 response during the acute response to viral infection. Additionally, this Th2 skewing may impair IL-10 production, which through its regulatory effects may help control the respiratory viral response in healthy individuals, but when deficient may contribute to RV-mediated exacerbations in asthmatic individuals.[54]

Respiratory viral infections often lead to asthma exacerbations several days after the initial viral inoculation. This is slower than asthma exacerbations from allergic stimuli but still rather rapid after the initial insult. Interestingly, there may be more similarity between respiratory viral infection-induced exacerbations and allergen-induced disease. In our mouse model of respiratory viral-induced asthma, the mice make IgE against SeV as early as day 3 after viral inoculation.[55] This IgE is necessary to lead to development of postviral airway disease, as we mentioned earlier. We use SeV to mimic the response to RSV, and intriguingly, there are several studies that demonstrate humans make IgE against RSV.[16,56-59] In fact, the level of IgE was correlated with the severity of the RSV-induced disease and subsequent wheezing.

We have demonstrated that humans make IgE against RV, suggesting that IgE against viruses may be part of the normal antiviral immune response.[17] If antiviral IgE did activate mast cells and lead to airway disease in a manner akin to an allergen-induced exacerbation,[60] then treatment with anti-IgE would be expected to prevent viral-induced asthma exacerbations. Indeed, treatment of children with anti-IgE led to the protection against asthma exacerbations not only in the spring and fall pollen season but also in the winter viral season.[61] In another study, treatment with anti-IgE before an experimental RV infection led to significantly reduced airway symptoms in the 4 days immediately following the viral inoculation.[62] This is similar to the timing of what we see in our mouse model (IgE seems early) but also suggests that IgE has its strongest effect during the innate immune response to the virus. These 2 studies thus suggest that virus-induced asthma exacerbations may be much more similar to other IgE-mediated exacerbations of the disease, where IgE cross-linking is associated with the activation of the innate immune response (mast cells or basophils, typically).

An alternative explanation for the success of anti-IgE in preventing viral-induced asthma exacerbations is related to the effect of IgE on plasmacytoid dendritic cells (PDCs). PDCs express abundant type I IFN, which is a potent antiviral, as well as FcεRI, the high affinity receptor for IgE. Cross-linking IgE on the surface of a PDC reduces the production of type I IFN, and it has been proposed that viral-induced asthma exacerbations are related to impaired type I IFN production in asthma patients.[63] One concern relates to how decreased type I IFN would drive an asthma exacerbation because there is not a clear mechanistic connection to airway hyperreactivity or mucous cell metaplasia. The prevailing idea is that decreased type I IFN would lead to reduced antiviral immunity, and the increased viral replication would then cause further airway damage and that would lead to an exacerbation. However, as mentioned above, a recent experimental RV infection study demonstrated the opposite—subjects with allergic disease or asthma both had lower levels of RV than healthy controls, despite the fact that the atopic subjects all had worse symptoms (and the asthma patients had asthma exacerbations).[64] Thus, the connection among IgE, type I IFN, and asthma exacerbations remains inconclusive.

Another potential relationship between IgE and asthma exacerbations relates to the finding that RV-induced exacerbations were more common during allergen seasons.

This has suggested to some investigators that there may be a feed-forward loop involving mast cells and IgE in viral-induced exacerbations.[65] In this hypothesis, allergen cross-links IgE on mast cells leading to IL13 production. The presence of RV infection provides a second "hit" to the epithelial cells that were T2 primed by mast cell IL13. This then leads to a feed-forward loop involving ILC2 produced IL13 and eosinophils, and the subsequent asthma exacerbation. In this scheme, use of anti-IgE would prevent the initial priming of the airway and thus inhibit RV-induced asthma exacerbations.

Clearly, IgE plays a major role in respiratory virus-induced asthma exacerbations (**Fig. 1**). However, whether the exacerbation is a result of simple virus cross-linking antiviral IgE, working through PDC, or priming the airway epithelium is something that awaits further research. Nonetheless, all of these hypotheses do support the use of anti-IgE to prevent viral-induced exacerbations. Given the ability of anti-IL4ra treatment to reduce IgE levels,[66] it is also intriguing to wonder if treatment with anti-IL4ra therapy would also be able to prevent viral-induced asthma exacerbations.

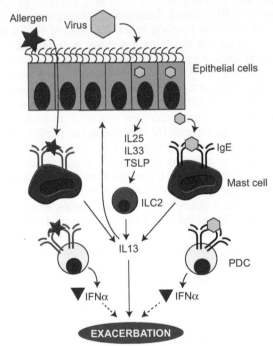

Fig. 1. Potential mechanisms for IgE-driven viral-induced asthma exacerbations. Allergen can cross-link allergen-specific IgE (red) on mast cells (*left side of panel*), which leads to IL13 production. This IL13 can prime the airway epithelial cells, so that a viral infection leads to the production of IL25, IL33, and TSLP. These cytokines recruit ILC2s, which produce IL13. This IL13 can feedback to the epithelia, as well as leading directly to an asthma exacerbation. Allergen-specific IgE can be cross-linked on PDCs, which reduces the amount of IFNα produced by the PDC and may contribute to the exacerbation. IgE against the virus itself may contribute directly to an asthma exacerbation (*right side of panel*), if this antiviral IgE (*blue*) is cross-linked by the virus. In this case, mast cells will produce IL13 (and other mediators) that can drive the exacerbation. Similarly, to the situation with allergen-specific IgE, cross-linking of antiviral IgE on PDC would also be predicted to reduce IFNα and further contribute to the exacerbation.

Indeed, post hoc evaluation of phase 3 data demonstrated a reduction in respiratory infection complaints in those treated with dupilumab compared with placebo.[67] Whether this is related to reduced IL4/13 directly or a reduction in IgE (against allergens or viruses) remains to be determined.

SUMMARY/DISCUSSION

This review has covered what the current thoughts are on how respiratory virus infection can lead to the development and exacerbation of asthma. As demonstrated above, the type and timing of viral infection is important, as well as the individual's underlying atopic status. Young infants are at risk of developing asthma (and atopy) with a severe RSV infection in the first 2 to 6 months of life, whereas RV will drive asthma development and exacerbation in those who already have developed an atopic predisposition. Further, it seems that the atopic immune response (ie, IgE and type 2 cytokines) is a component of the antiviral immune response (indeed, some think the atopic immune response may have developed as part of the antiviral response). This may be a reason for the intricate interaction between respiratory viral infection and asthma. Mouse models have informed us on several pathways that may be involved but it is human studies that have demonstrated potential roles for various mediators and IgE in viral-induced asthma exacerbations. The future is bright for continued investigation into the exquisite interplay among respiratory viruses, type 2 cytokines, IgE, and asthma development and exacerbation.

CLINICS CARE POINTS

- Respiratory syncytial virus (RSV) in early life increases the risk of wheezing and is associated with the development of asthma.
  - RSV lower respiratory tract infection in children aged younger than 3 years was associated with an increased risk of infrequent wheeze (OR 3.2) and frequent wheeze (OR 4.3) by age 6.
  - In the Avon Longitudinal Study of Parents and Children, children admitted to the hospital in the first 12 months of life with RSV bronchiolitis had a cumulative prevalence of asthma of 38.4% at 91 months of age, compared with 20.1% in the control group.[68]
- For patients with preexisting allergic disease, rhinovirus infections induce wheezing and cause exacerbations of asthma.
  - Allergic sensitization led to an increased risk of wheezing caused by human RV but not RSV.[69]
  - Children with human RV bronchiolitis with wheezing in the first year of life were more likely to have persistent wheeze at 10 years.[61,70]
  - In most cases, asthma exacerbations will start within a few days of the viral infection. Viral infections cause an increase in airway hyperresponsiveness during the time of peak virus symptoms, and these changes can last for several weeks.[71] Anti-IgE seems to be effective in preventing viral-induced asthma exacerbations; however, the actual mechanism by which it does is not fully defined and remains controversial.
  - Omalizumab reduced the proportion of patients who had one or more exacerbations during a 60-week period from 49% to 30% but omalizumab does not prevent the viral infection itself. Two possible mechanisms for the effect of omalizumab include a decrease in damaged epithelium that results from underlying allergic inflammation[72] and the prevention of IgE-dependent immune responses that may interfere with antiviral immune responses.[63]
- It remains to be seen if therapies that block IL-4, IL5, or IL-13 pathways reduce viral-induced exacerbations but there are rationales that would support these approaches. For now, we await clinical studies.

Th2 cytokines, such as IL-4, IL-5, and IL-13, inhibit antiviral defense pathways, with examples including inhibition of toll like receptor 3 (TLR3) and interferon regulatory factor 3 (IRF3).[73]
o It is plausible that normalizing Th1 and Th2 cytokine patterns could reduce the risk of viral respiratory infections, and this could reduce the risk of virus-induced asthma exacerbations but this is yet to be elucidated.

DISCLOSURE

M.H. Grayson is the Editor-in-Chief of the Annals of Allergy, Asthma & Immunology; has served on advisory boards for AbbVie, GSK, and Merck; has stock options in Invirsa, Inc.; serves on the Board of Directors of the American Board of Allergy and Immunology, Asthma and Allergy Foundation of America (AAFA), where he is Chair of their Medical Scientific Council; and is a member of the American Lung Association Scientific Advisory Committee. The other authors have no conflicts to declare.

REFERENCES

1. Asthma- Level 3 cause. Lancet 2020;396.
2. Most Recent National Asthma Data. Center for Disease Control and Prevention. 2022. Available at: https://www.cdc.gov/asthma/most_recent_national_asthma_data.htm. Accessed June 6, 2022.
3. Nurmagambetov T, Kuwahara R, Garbe P. The Economic Burden of Asthma in the United States, 2008-2013. Ann Am Thorac Soc 2018;15(3):348–56.
4. Pawelczyk M, Kowalski ML. The Role of Human Parainfluenza Virus Infections in the Immunopathology of the Respiratory Tract. Curr Allergy Asthma Rep 2017; 17(3):16.
5. Jackson DJ, Gern JE, Lemanske RF Jr. The contributions of allergic sensitization and respiratory pathogens to asthma inception. J Allergy Clin Immunol 2016; 137(3):659–65 [quiz: 66].
6. Resiliac J, Grayson MH. Epidemiology of Infections and Development of Asthma. Immunol Allergy Clin North Am 2019;39(3):297–307.
7. Wu P, Hartert TV. Evidence for a causal relationship between respiratory syncytial virus infection and asthma. Expert Rev Anti Infect Ther 2011;9(9):731–45.
8. Shay DK, Holman RC, Newman RD, et al. Bronchiolitis-associated hospitalizations among US children, 1980-1996. JAMA 1999;282(15):1440–6.
9. Wos M, Sanak M, Soja J, et al. The presence of rhinovirus in lower airways of patients with bronchial asthma. Am J Respir Crit Care Med 2008;177(10):1082–9.
10. Cheung DS, Grayson MH. Role of viruses in the development of atopic disease in pediatric patients. Curr Allergy Asthma Rep 2012;12(6):613–20.
11. Mikhail I, Grayson MH. Asthma and viral infections: An intricate relationship. Ann Allergy Asthma Immunol 2019;123(4):352–8.
12. Meissner HC. Viral Bronchiolitis in Children. N Engl J Med 2016;374(1):62–72.
13. Cheung DS, Ehlenbach SJ, Kitchens RT, et al. Cutting edge: CD49d+ neutrophils induce FcepsilonRI expression on lung dendritic cells in a mouse model of post-viral asthma. J Immunol 2010;185(9):4983–7.
14. Sigua JA, Buelow B, Cheung DS, et al. CD49d-expressing neutrophils differentiate atopic from nonatopic individuals. J Allergy Clin Immunol 2014;133(3): 901–4.e5.

15. Subrata LS, Bizzintino J, Mamessier E, et al. Interactions between innate antiviral and atopic immunoinflammatory pathways precipitate and sustain asthma exacerbations in children. J Immunol 2009;183(4):2793–800.

16. Khan SH, Grayson MH. Cross-linking IgE augments human conventional dendritic cell production of CC chemokine ligand 28. J Allergy Clin Immunol 2010; 125(1):265–7.

17. Tam JS, Jackson WT, Hunter D, et al. Rhinovirus specific IgE can be detected in human sera. J Allergy Clin Immunol 2013;132(5):1241–3.

18. Tam JS, Grayson MH. IgE and antiviral immune response in asthma. J Allergy Clin Immunol 2017;139(5):1717.

19. Bui RH, Molinaro GA, Kettering JD, et al. Virus-specific IgE and IgG4 antibodies in serum of children infected with respiratory syncytial virus. J Pediatr 1987; 110(1):87–90.

20. Rabatic S, Gagro A, Lokar-Kolbas R, et al. Increase in CD23+ B cells in infants with bronchiolitis is accompanied by appearance of IgE and IgG4 antibodies specific for respiratory syncytial virus. J Infect Dis 1997;175(1):32–7.

21. Miura TA. Respiratory epithelial cells as master communicators during viral infections. Curr Clin Microbiol Rep 2019;6(1):10–7.

22. Land W. Role of DAMPs in respiratory virus-induced acute respiratory distress syndrome—with a preliminary reference to SARS-CoV-2 pneumonia. Genes Immun 2021;22:141–60.

23. Vareille M, Kieninger E, Edwards MR, et al. The airway epithelium: soldier in the fight against respiratory viruses. Clin Microbiol Rev 2011;24(1):210–29.

24. Buchweitz JP, Harkema JR, Kaminski NE. Time-dependent airway epithelial and inflammatory cell responses induced by influenza virus A/PR/8/34 in C57BL/6 mice. Toxicol Pathol 2007;35(3):424–35.

25. Munitz A, Brandt EB, Mingler M, et al. Distinct roles for IL-13 and IL-4 via IL-13 receptor alpha1 and the type II IL-4 receptor in asthma pathogenesis. Proc Natl Acad Sci U S A 2008;105(20):7240–5.

26. Stier MT, Bloodworth MH, Toki S, et al. Respiratory syncytial virus infection activates IL-13-producing group 2 innate lymphoid cells through thymic stromal lymphopoietin. J Allergy Clin Immunol 2016;138(3):814–24.e11.

27. Lee HC, Headley MB, Loo YM, et al. Thymic stromal lymphopoietin is induced by respiratory syncytial virus-infected airway epithelial cells and promotes a type 2 response to infection. J Allergy Clin Immunol 2012;130(5):1187–96.e5.

28. Han M, Rajput C, Hong JY, et al. The Innate Cytokines IL-25, IL-33, and TSLP Cooperate in the Induction of Type 2 Innate Lymphoid Cell Expansion and Mucous Metaplasia in Rhinovirus-Infected Immature Mice. J Immunol 2017;199(4): 1308–18.

29. Watson B, Gauvreau GM. Thymic stromal lymphopoietin: a central regulator of allergic asthma. Expert Opin Ther Targets 2014;18(7):771–85.

30. Saenz SA, Taylor BC, Artis D. Welcome to the neighborhood: epithelial cell-derived cytokines license innate and adaptive immune responses at mucosal sites. Immunol Rev 2008;226:172–90.

31. Camelo A, Guglielmo R, Oea Y. IL-33, IL-25, and TSLP induce a distinct phenotypic and activation profile in human type 2 innate lymphoid cells. Blood Adv 2017;1(10):577–89.

32. Sastre B, Garcia-Garcia ML, Canas JA, et al. Bronchiolitis and recurrent wheezing are distinguished by type 2 innate lymphoid cells and immune response. Pediatr Allergy Immunol 2021;32(1):51–9.

33. Jackson DJ, Makrinioti H, Rana BM, et al. IL-33-dependent type 2 inflammation during rhinovirus-induced asthma exacerbations in vivo. Am J Respir Crit Care Med 2014;190(12):1373–82.

34. Borish L, Feng X, Mea R. Reduced innate immunity in asthma compensated by enhanced anti-viral type 2 responses against experimental rhinovirus (RV) inoculation. J Allergy Clin Immunol 2020;145(2). https://doi.org/10.1016/j.jaci.2019.12.355.

35. Hossain FMA, Choi JY, Uyangaa E, et al. The Interplay between Host Immunity and Respiratory Viral Infection in Asthma Exacerbation. Immune Netw 2019;19(5):e31.

36. Taveras J, Garcia-Maurino C, Moore-Clingenpeel M. The Protective Role of Mucosal Interferons in Infants with Respiratory Syncytial Virus (RSV) Infection. Open Forum Infect Dis 2020;7(1):195–6.

37. Edwards M, Regamey N, Mea V. Impaired innate interferon induction in severe therapy resistant atopic asthmatic children. Mucosal Immunol 2013;6:797–806.

38. Pitrez PM, Brennan S, Sly PD. Inflammatory profile in nasal secretions of infants hospitalized with acute lower airway tract infections. Respirology 2005;10(3):365–70.

39. Johnston SL. Innate immunity in the pathogenesis of virus-induced asthma exacerbations. Proc Am Thorac Soc 2007;4(3):267–70.

40. Garcia C, Soriano-Fallas A, Lozano J, et al. Decreased innate immune cytokine responses correlate with disease severity in children with respiratory syncytial virus and human rhinovirus bronchiolitis. Pediatr Infect Dis J 2012;31(1):86–9.

41. Johnston SL, Pattemore PK, Sanderson G, et al. Community study of role of viral infections in exacerbations of asthma in 9-11 year old children. BMJ 1995;310(6989):1225–9.

42. Friedlander SL, Busse WW. The role of rhinovirus in asthma exacerbations. J Allergy Clin Immunol 2005;116(2):267–73.

43. Khetsuriani N, Kazerouni NN, Erdman DD, et al. Prevalence of viral respiratory tract infections in children with asthma. J Allergy Clin Immunol 2007;119(2):314–21.

44. Gern JE. Viral and bacterial infections in the development and progression of asthma. J Allergy Clin Immunol 2000;105(2 Pt 2):S497–502.

45. Denlinger LC, Sorkness RL, Lee WM, et al. Lower airway rhinovirus burden and the seasonal risk of asthma exacerbation. Am J Respir Crit Care Med 2011;184(9):1007–14.

46. Adeli M, El-Shareif T, Hendaus MA. Asthma exacerbation related to viral infections: An up to date summary. J Fam Med Prim Care 2019;8(9):2753–9.

47. Zheng SY, Wang LL, Ren L, et al. Epidemiological analysis and follow-up of human rhinovirus infection in children with asthma exacerbation. J Med Virol 2018;90(2):219–28.

48. Bizzintino J, Lee WM, Laing IA, et al. Association between human rhinovirus C and severity of acute asthma in children. Eur Respir J 2011;37(5):1037–42.

49. Medzhitov R. Origin and physiological roles of inflammation. Nature 2008;454(7203):428–35.

50. Stenfeldt AL, Wenneras C. Danger signals derived from stressed and necrotic epithelial cells activate human eosinophils. Immunology 2004;112(4):605–14.

51. Weng Q, Zhu C, Zheng K, et al. Early recruited neutrophils promote asthmatic inflammation exacerbation by release of neutrophil elastase. Cell Immunol 2020;352:104101.

52. Cardell LO, Agusti C, Takeyama K, et al. LTB(4)-induced nasal gland serous cell secretion mediated by neutrophil elastase. Am J Respir Crit Care Med 1999; 160(2):411–4.

53. Sun LH, Chen AH, Yang ZF, et al. Respiratory syncytial virus induces leukotriene C4 synthase expression in bronchial epithelial cells. Respirology 2013;18(Suppl 3):40–6.

54. Message SD, Laza-Stanca V, Mallia P, et al. Rhinovirus-induced lower respiratory illness is increased in asthma and related to virus load and Th1/2 cytokine and IL-10 production. Proc Natl Acad Sci U S A 2008;105(36):13562–7.

55. Grayson MH, Cheung D, Rohlfing MM, et al. Induction of high-affinity IgE receptor on lung dendritic cells during viral infection leads to mucous cell metaplasia. J Exp Med 2007;204(11):2759–69.

56. Robert C, Welliver MS, Rinaldo D, et al. Respiratory Syncytial Virus-Specific IgE Responses following Infection: Evidence for a Predominantly Mucosal Response. Pediatr Res 1985;19(5):420–4.

57. Martorano LM, Grayson MH. Respiratory viral infections and atopic development: From possible mechanisms to advances in treatment. Eur J Immunol 2018;48(3): 407–14.

58. Sigurs N, Bjarnason R, Sigurbergsson F, et al. Asthma and immunoglobulin E antibodies after respiratory syncytial virus bronchiolitis: a prospective cohort study with matched controls. Pediatrics 1995;95(4):500–5.

59. Vasudev M, Cheung DS, Pincsak H, et al. Expression of high-affinity IgE receptor on human peripheral blood dendritic cells in children. PLoS One 2012;7(2): e32556.

60. Chen CH, Lin YT, Yang YH, et al. Ribavirin for respiratory syncytial virus bronchiolitis reduced the risk of asthma and allergen sensitization. Pediatr Allergy Immunol 2008;19(2):166–72.

61. Busse WW, Morgan WJ, Gergen PJ, et al. Randomized trial of omalizumab (anti-IgE) for asthma in inner-city children. N Engl J Med 2011;364(11):1005–15.

62. Heymann PW, Platts-Mills TAE, Woodfolk JA, et al. Understanding the asthmatic response to an experimental rhinovirus infection: Exploring the effects of blocking IgE. J Allergy Clin Immunol 2020;146(3):545–54.

63. Gill MA, Bajwa G, George TA, et al. Counterregulation between the FcepsilonRI pathway and antiviral responses in human plasmacytoid dendritic cells. J Immunol 2010;184(11):5999–6006.

64. Feng X, Lawrence MG, Payne SC, et al. Lower viral loads in subjects with rhinovirus-challenged allergy despite reduced innate immunity. Ann Allergy Asthma Immunol 2022;128(4):414–422 e2.

65. Larry Borish M. Rethinking the central role of mast cells in virally mediated asthma exacerbations. Ann Allergy Asthma Immunol 2022. https://doi.org/10.1016/j.anai.2022.03.029.

66. William W, Busse M. Efficacy of dupilumab on clinical outcomes in patients with asthma and perennial allergic rhinitis. Ann Allergy Asthma Immunol 2020;125(5): 565–76.

67. Geng Mea B. Respiratory Infections and Anti-Infective Medication Use From Phase 3 Dupilumab Respiratory Studies. J Allergy Clin Immunol Pract 2021; 10(3):732–41.

68. Henderson J, Hilliard TN, Sherriff A, et al. Hospitalization for RSV bronchiolitis before 12 months of age and subsequent asthma, atopy and wheeze: a longitudinal birth cohort study. Pediatr Allergy Immunol 2005;16(5):386–92.

69. Jackson DJ, Evans MD, Gangnon RE, et al. Evidence for a causal relationship between allergic sensitization and rhinovirus wheezing in early life. Am J Respir Crit Care Med 2012;185(3):281–5.
70. Kusel MM, Kebadze T, Johnston SL, et al. Febrile respiratory illnesses in infancy and atopy are risk factors for persistent asthma and wheeze. Eur Respir J 2012; 39(4):876–82.
71. Gern JE. Viral respiratory infection and the link to asthma. Pediatr Infect Dis J 2004;23(1 Suppl):S78–86.
72. Jakiela B, Brockman-Schneider R, Amineva S, et al. Basal cells of differentiated bronchial epithelium are more susceptible to rhinovirus infection. Am J Respir Cell Mol Biol 2008;38(5):517–23.
73. Contoli M, Ito K, Padovani A, et al. Th2 cytokines impair innate immune responses to rhinovirus in respiratory epithelial cells. Allergy 2015;70(8):910–20.

Viral Infections and Wheezing in Preschool Children

Alexa M.A. Doss, MD*, Jeffrey R. Stokes, MD[1]

KEYWORDS

- Wheezing • Asthma • Preschool • Viral infection

KEY POINTS

- Wheezing is common in childhood with approximately 50% of children experiencing at least 1 wheezing episode within their first 6 years of life while only 8% of children have asthma.
- Lower lung function, in children who wheeze, is set by 6 years of life.
- Respiratory syncytial virus (RSV) and rhinovirus account for most viruses detected in children with RSV causing the most wheezing episodes in children aged less than 1 year. Rhinovirus causes more wheezing episodes in children aged 1 year and older.
- Asthma indices can help predict which wheezing children will develop asthma.
- Inhaled corticosteroids (ICS) are commonly used to treat wheezing in preschool children. Both intermittent and daily ICS can be used. The effectiveness of oral corticosteroids in this age range is inconclusive.

INTRODUCTION

Wheezing is common in childhood; approximately 50% of children will have at least one wheezing episode in their first 6 years of life, yet only 8% of children will develop asthma.[1] Respiratory viral infections are triggers for childhood wheezing with respiratory syncytial virus (RSV) and rhinovirus being the 2 most common infections to cause wheezing in early childhood.[2] Children with viral-induced wheezing comprise a cohort that can go on to develop asthma.

Asthma is chronic, high morbidity disease which requires long-term medical management. In childhood, there is a male predominance of asthma diagnoses in children aged 0–9 years, yet the reverse is observed in late adolescence through adulthood.[3,4] Up to 60% of asthmatic children have at least one asthma exacerbation per year.[4,5]

Division of Pediatric Allergy, Immunology, and Pulmonary Medicine, St. Louis Children's Hospital, St Louis, MO, USA
[1] Present address: 6170 Kingsbury Avenue, Saint Louis, MO 63112.
* Corresponding author. 1 Children's Place, CB 8116, Saint Louis, MO 63110.
E-mail address: alexa.altman@wustl.edu

Immunol Allergy Clin N Am 42 (2022) 727–741
https://doi.org/10.1016/j.iac.2022.05.004
0889-8561/22/© 2022 Elsevier Inc. All rights reserved.

Children with asthma aged 0 to 4 years have the highest rate of asthma-related health care visits, accounting for twice the rate of emergency department (ED) visits and 3 times the rate of hospitalizations compared with adolescents with asthma.[5,6] In addition to health care visits and hospitalizations, approximately 50% of school-aged asthmatics are absent from one or more day of school per year.[6]

WHEEZING PHENOTYPES

Multiple wheezing phenotypes have been identified in childhood. Classifying these wheezing phenotypes helps guide management and identifies the children who will experience future wheezing episodes. The Tuscan Children's Respiratory Study (TCRS) prospectively followed 1246 newborns and defined 4 childhood wheezing phenotypes: never wheeze (no wheezing episodes, 51.5%), transient early wheeze (wheezing episodes that stopped after age 3 years, 19.9%), late-onset wheeze (first wheezing episode after age 4 years, 15%), and persistent wheeze (wheezing episodes beginning before age 3 years and persisted, 13.7%).[1] The TCRS saw that patterns of lung function and atopy by age 6 years persisted through age 16 years with children who had higher atopy and immunoglobulin E (IgE) levels in the late-onset wheezers and persistent wheezers.[7] Additionally, lower lung function seen in the transient early wheezers and persistent wheezers at age 6 also persisted through age 16.[7] The TCRS results indicate that the lung function deficits detected in children with asthma are present by age 6 years and not due to their ongoing disease process.[1]

The Prevention and Incidence of Asthma and Mite Allergy (PIAMA) study used latent class analysis to identify respiratory phenotypes in 2810 participants from the Netherlands birth cohort.[8] In addition to the 4 phenotypes identified by the TCRS and described above, the PIAMA study identified a fifth phenotype of intermediate-onset wheeze (onset of wheeze after age 2 years and persisted).[8] The Avon Longitudinal Study of Parents and Children (ALSPAC) study also used latent class analysis to evaluate 6265 United Kingdom birth cohort participants and, in addition to those phenotypes found in the TCRS and PIAMA study, identified a sixth phenotype of prolonged early wheeze (wheezing episodes that stopped at age 5 years).[9] The ALSPAC study evaluated lung function at 24 years of age and found lower lung function in the persistent wheeze and transient-early wheeze compared with the never wheeze phenotype as also shown with the TCRS cohort.[10] Both the ALSPAC and PIAMA study showed the intermediate-onset, late-onset, and persistent wheeze phenotypes were strongly associated with indoor allergen sensitization seen by age 4 years.[8]

The Childhood Asthma Research and Education (CARE) Network identified 4 phenotypes based on atopy and wheezing from 1708 preschool children: (1) minimal sensitization (30%), (2) sensitization with indoor pet exposure (25%), (3) sensitization with tobacco smoke exposure (25%) and (4) multiple sensitizations plus eczema (20%).[11] The probability of wheezing per 2-year period was highest in groups 2 and 4.[11] As CARE had data from 5 clinic trials, treatment response was available and showed that daily inhaled corticosteroids (ICS) improved the frequency of exacerbations in groups 2 and 4 only.[11] The Urban Environment and Childhood Asthma birth cohort prospectively evaluated 442 inner city children and identified 5 phenotypes: (1) low wheeze/low atopy (26%), (2) low wheeze/high atopy (18%), (3) transient wheeze/low atopy (17%), (4) high wheeze/low atopy (23%), and (5) high wheeze/high atopy (15%).[12] Indoor allergen exposure in the first year of life differed in the high and low wheezing phenotypes with the 2 high wheezing phenotypes having the lowest cumulative exposure to indoor allergens.[12] Asthma rates were greatest in high wheezing/high atopy and high wheezing/low atopy, at 70% and 67%, respectively. Children exhibiting the high wheezing/high atopy phenotype also had the greatest lung function impairment.[12]

CHILDHOOD VIRAL INFECTIONS

Viral infections are common among children; the average child will contract 6 to 8 viral infections per year, with increasing rates if the child attends daycare.[13] Wheezing episodes are frequently triggered by respiratory viral infections.[13,14] Viruses have been detected in 80% to 90% of children with wheeze and cough compared with 21% of healthy, asymptomatic children.[2,14–16] RSV and rhinovirus, the most commonly detected viral pathogens with wheezing illnesses, account for 69% of all detected viral infections within the first 3 years of life.[2] Children who wheezed with RSV and/or rhinovirus at ages 0 to 3 years had an increased risk of asthma at age 6.[17] The Childhood Origins of Asthma (COAST) prospective birth cohort of 289 newborns noted that children who wheezed with rhinovirus had nearly a 10-fold increase in wheezing by age 3 years, whereas children with RSV-induced wheezing were 2.6 times more likely to have wheezing by age 3 years.[17]

RHINOVIRUS

Rhinovirus is the most common virus to cause wheezing in children aged 1 year and older.[14,18] Rhinoviruses (Enterovirus genus, Picornaviridae family) are classified into 3 species: A, B, and C.[18] Rhinovirus A and C cause more severe illness in infants than B.[18] Wheezing with rhinovirus infection is a strong predictor of future wheezing episodes, and this prediction is higher in atopic individuals.[14,17] A cross-sectional emergency department (ED) study of 70 children presenting with wheezing showed most wheezing episodes were in children aged 2 to 16 years with rhinovirus infection and evidence of atopy or eosinophilic airway inflammation.[14] Similar results were seen in the Childhood Asthma Study (CAS) prospective cohort of 234 Australian children at high risk for developing atopic disease.[16] Preschool children wheezing with rhinovirus-C infection had 7 times greater risk of wheezing at age 5 and 10 years if atopic by 2 years of age compared with nonatopic children. Genetics, such as 17q21 variants are associated with rhinovirus wheezing in childhood and an increased risk of asthma.[19]

RESPIRATORY SYNCYTIAL VIRUS

RSV is the most common viral infection in infants younger than 1 year to cause wheezing.[18] RSV (Orthopneumovirus genus and the Paramyxoviradae family) has 2 main antigenic groups, A and B with RSV-A causes more severe illness.[18] Although RSV is the leading cause of hospitalization in infants aged younger than 1 year in the United States, most RSV infections are mild or asymptomatic.[18,20] RSV is the most prominent virus to cause wheezing in infancy; however, it is not significant in adolescents. The TCRS reported that the prevalence of RSV lower respiratory tract illnesses before age 3 years was associated with a significant increase in risk of subsequent wheezing during the first 10 years but was not significant by age 13.[21]

Palivizumab is a monoclonal antibody given to high-risk infants to prevent severe RSV infection.[22] In the Netherlands, 429 otherwise healthy preterm infants (33–35 weeks estimated gestational age) were enrolled in a double-blind, placebo-controlled trial to receive palivizumab or placebo during RSV season.[22] In the first year of life, the palivizumab cohort had a 61% relative risk reduction of total wheezing days compared with placebo.[22] The percentage of physician-diagnosed asthma was similar between the 2 groups: 10% of those treated with palivizumab and 9.9% with placebo.[23] There was no statistical significant difference in lung function between the 2 groups.[23]

Both viral-induced wheezing and aeroallergen sensitization are risk factors for asthma development in childhood. The COAST birth cohort study sought to determine the developmental sequence for asthma diagnosis.[2] This was a prospective, birth-cohort of 285 children at high risk for allergic disease and asthma followed through 13 years of age.[2,24] Children who were sensitized to aeroallergens had a greater risk of developing viral wheeze than nonsensitized children.[2] Additionally, the earlier in life sensitization occurred, the higher the rate of asthma at age 13.[24] This study demonstrated that allergic sensitization precedes rhinovirus wheezing and that viral wheezing did not increase the likelihood of developing allergic sensitization.[2]

CHILDHOOD BACTERIAL INFECTIONS

In addition to viral infections, airway bacteria can also influence the development of asthma.[18] Upper airway bacteria colonization is common, and the colonized species can influence wheeze in childhood.[20] The most common bacterium found in upper airways in childhood include *Staphylococcus, Streptococcus, Moraxella, Haemophilus, Dolosigranulum,* and *Corynebacterium*.[20] In children aged 0 to 3 years, pathogenic bacteria have been identified in 86% of wheezing episodes with 31% of episodes without viral detection.[25] Although certain bacterial pathogens are associated with wheezing and asthma, a diverse airway microbiome can be protective against wheezing illnesses.[18] Many studies have demonstrated colonization with *S. pneumoniae, M. catarrhalis,* and *H. influenzae* in infants are associated with an increased incidence of recurrent wheezing and asthma in childhood, whereas *Corynebacterium, Staphylococcus,* and *Dolosigranulum* are more often found in the absence of respiratory symptoms and viral detection.[18,26]

Bacterial colonization before the first upper respiratory infection influences the development of asthma.[16,27] The CAS prospective birth cohort of 234 Australian children at high risk for atopic disease were evaluated for bacteria and viruses when asymptomatic at scheduled screenings and with respiratory illness.[16] Infants who had early asymptomatic colonization with *Streptococcus* were subject to an increased risk of asthma 3-fold to 4-fold.[16]

Because bacteria and viruses are so prevalent in childhood, studies have evaluated the effects of different bacterial and viral combinations. Cross-sectional cohort studies have demonstrated increased *Moraxella* and *Haemophilus* in rhinovirus bronchiolitis, whereas RSV bronchiolitis had increased *Streptococcus* and *Haemophilus* species.[20] Rhinovirus and *S. pneumoniae* detection was associated with increased moderate asthma exacerbations.[27] In the absence of rhinovirus, *S. pneumoniae* was associated with increased upper respiratory symptoms and moderate asthma exacerbations.[27]

PREDICTING ASTHMA IN CHILDHOOD

Although there are many wheezing infants, it is difficult to know from their clinical presentation who will develop asthma. Additionally, there is not a single biomarker to predict which children will develop asthma.[28] Predictive indices are useful in prospectively identifying those infants at risk to develop asthma and distinguishing them from the transient wheezers. The initial asthma predictive index (API) was established using data from the TCRS.[28] The API has been modified (mAPI) and used in clinical trials for the CARE network.[29] A positive mAPI is defined as 4 or more wheezing

> **Box 1**
> **Modified asthma predictive index**
>
> - A history of 4 or more wheezing episodes in the last year with at least one that was physician-diagnosed
> - Must meet 1 major or 2 minor conditions
>
> Major Criteria
> - Parental history of asthma
> - Physician-diagnosed atopic dermatitis
> - Allergic sensitization to at least 1 aeroallergen
>
> Minor Criteria
> - Allergic sensitization to milk, egg, or peanut
> - Wheezing unrelated to colds
> - Blood eosinophils ≥4%

episodes in the prior year with at least 1 physician-diagnosed event accompanied with either 1 major or 2 minor criteria (**Box 1**). Major criteria for the mAPI include parental history of asthma, physician-diagnosed atopic dermatitis, or allergic sensitization to at least 1 aeroallergen. Minor criteria include allergic sensitization to milk, egg, or peanut, wheezing unrelated to colds, and blood eosinophilia 4% or greater. The mAPI has high a posttest probability at 72% for unselected populations and 90% in high-risk populations.[30]

The Pediatric Asthma Risk Score (PARS) used data from the Cincinnati Childhood Allergy and Air Pollution study birth cohort of 762 children and identified 6 risk factors in children at age 3 years to predict asthma development at age 7 years (**Table 1**).[31] In addition to parental asthma, atopic dermatitis, and wheezing unrelated to colds as identified in the API, risk factors included early wheezing, sensitization to 2 or more food allergens or aeroallergens, and African American race.[31] PARS is a more effective system for predicting mild-to-moderate asthma compared with the API as children with mild asthma commonly have fewer risk factors and do not meet the API criteria.[31]

Table 1
Pediatric asthma risk score

Yes/No Question	Point Value	Total Score	Risk of Asthma by Age 7
Parental Asthma	2	0–4	3%–11%
Eczema by Age 3	2		
Early Wheezing by Age 3	3	5–8	15%–32%
Wheezing when Healthy	3		
African Ancestry	2	9–14	40%–79%
Positive SPT to ≥2 Food or Aeroallergen	2		

Abbreviation: SPT, skin prick test.

TREATMENT
Daily Inhaled Corticosteroids

ICS are effective in reducing the risk of asthma exacerbations in school-aged children, adolescents, and adults. As such, multiple trials have evaluated ICS in preschool-aged children. The Preventing Early Asthma in Kids (PEAK) trial was a double-blind, randomized, placebo-controlled, parallel group comparison of daily inhaled fluticasone propionate with placebo in 285 children aged 2 to 3 years with a positive mAPI.[29] PEAK was designed to evaluate the efficacy of daily ICS use during a 2 year period and its effect preventing high-risk children from developing asthma.[29] Children on daily ICS had more episode-free days, fewer exacerbations, and decreased use of other controlled medications compared with children receiving placebo.[29] A 1 year observation period followed the 2 year treatment period. At the end of the observation year, there were no differences in the number of exacerbations, episode-free days, or lung function in the 2 groups.[29] Even though the use of ICS did not prevent asthma, it demonstrated patients who benefited from daily ICS: male sex, Caucasian, history of ED visit or hospitalization for asthma within the prior year, aeroallergen sensitization, and less than 80% episode-free days during the run-in period.[29]

The Individualized Therapy for Asthma in Toddlers (INFANT) study was a randomized, double-blind, double-dummy clinical trial in 300 children aged 12 to 59 months with asthma requiring treatment with daily controller.[32] The study included 3 crossover periods consisting of daily ICS, daily leukotriene receptor antagonists (LTRAs), and as-needed ICS treatment coadministered with albuterol.[32] Seventy-four percent of the participants had a differential response to the 3 treatments with approximately 50% having the best response to daily ICS and 25% each with the best response to intermittent ICS or daily LTRA.[32] Factors that predicted best control with daily ICS included aeroallergen sensitization and blood eosinophil count of 300/mL or greater.[32] Additionally, serum eosinophilic cation protein levels of 10 mg/L or greater and sensitization to dog and/or cat predicted greater daily ICS response. The children without differential response had less disease activity.[32] Serum IgE levels and mAPI status did not influence a differential response pattern. No factors were noted for improved response to as-needed ICS or LTRA.[32]

Papi and colleagues[33] performed a randomized, parallel-group, three-group, double-blind, double-dummy, placebo-controlled study in 276 children aged 1 to 4 years with frequent wheeze randomized to receive daily ICS and as-needed short-acting beta agonist (SABA), daily placebo and as-needed ICS + SABA, or daily placebo and SABA. The daily ICS cohort exhibited the greatest number of symptom-free days at 70%, followed by as-needed ICS + SABA at 65%, and the SABA only group having the least number of symptom-free days at 61%.[33] There was a greater time to first exacerbation in the daily ICS group with no difference in time to first exacerbation in the 2 remaining groups.

Kaiser and colleagues[34] performed a meta-analysis using 15 studies of daily ICS versus placebo showing an overall reduction in exacerbation rate with daily ICS compared with placebo at 12.9% and 24.0%, respectively. They estimated that the treatment of 9 children would prevent an asthma exacerbation in 1 child.[34] Studies have examined increasing the ICS dose at the onset of acute exacerbation in patients adherent to daily ICS and found no difference in the rate of exacerbations requiring treatment with systemic corticosteroids compared with maintaining standard daily ICS.[35] This does not hold true for children who are not taking daily ICS and benefits have been observed in starting ICS at the onset of symptoms as discussed below.

Intermittent Inhaled Corticosteroids

Many preschool children only wheeze with viral infections and are symptom free between episodes. Given this pattern, intermittent ICS has been studied to evaluate the efficacy of as-needed therapy compared with daily ICS. The Maintenance and Intermittent Inhaled Corticosteroids in Wheezing Toddlers (MIST) trial enrolled 278 children aged 12 to 53 months with a positive mAPI and recurrent wheezing episodes (at least 1 in the 12 months before the trials) in a randomized, double-blind, parallel group study.[36] Treatment groups included intermittent, high-dose budesonide for 7 days at the start of symptom onset or daily, low-dose budesonide with corresponding placebos.[36] There was no significant difference in the number of exacerbations requiring systemic corticosteroids, time to first or second exacerbation, or treatment failures between the groups.[36] The mean ICS exposure was 69% less in the intermittent regimen than daily regimen, 46 mg versus 150 mg, respectively.[36]

The Prevention of Asthma in Childhood study enrolled 411 1-month-old infants of asthmatic mothers in a double-blind, randomized, placebo control trial.[37] Treatment consisted of budesonide or placebo given for 2 weeks after a 3 day episode of wheezing. No statistical differences were seen in the number of symptom-free days, duration of acute episodes, or persistent wheezing between the 2 groups.[37]

Ducharme and colleagues[38] performed a randomized, parallel-group, placebo-controlled trial with triple blinding in 5 institutions in Quebec in 129 children aged 1 to 6 years to receive as-needed ICS versus placebo.[38] Participants were required to have 3 or more wheezing episodes in their lifetime. The children were randomized to ICS twice daily for 10 days at the onset of upper respiratory tract infection or placebo.[38] At the end of the 6 to 12 months treatment period, the ICS cohort required less treatment with systemic corticosteroids, 8% in the treatment group compared with 18% in placebo.[38] A statistically significant difference was observed in height with greater slowing of height in the treatment group at 6.23 cm compared with 6.56 cm in the placebo cohort.[38]

Kaiser and colleagues[34] meta-analysis of 5 studies involving 422 participants aged 6 years or younger treating with intermittent high-dose ICS with intermittent asthma or recurrent viral-triggered wheezing reduced the risk of exacerbation by 35% compared with placebo. They estimated that the treatment of 6 children will prevent an asthma exacerbation in 1 child.[34] In meta-analysis of 2 studies comparing daily ICS to intermittent ICS in 498 children with ages ranging 12 to 59 months, there was no difference in rates of severe exacerbation.[34] When deciding treatment of daily versus intermittent ICS preschool children with persistent symptoms, elevated blood eosinophils or aeroallergen sensitization benefited from daily ICS over intermittent treatment. Those children who had no wheezing episodes between respiratory infections, who are male, Caucasian, and visited the ED or were hospitalized in the past year due to wheezing or have aeroallergen sensitization, may have greater benefit from daily ICS. In all other children aged 5 years and younger, intermittent ICS should be sufficient.

Leukotriene Receptor Antagonists

Valovirta and colleagues[39] evaluated 1771 patients aged 6 months to 5 years in a double-blind, double-dummy, parallel group study randomized to receive daily montelukast, intermittent montelukast, or placebo in a 52-week study. Enrollment requirements included episodes of asthma symptoms in the preceding year that required SABA treatment, at least 1 treatment with oral corticosteroids (OCS) or hospitalization for asthma with asymptomatic periods between episodes. There were no significant differences in the daily versus intermittent montelukast group compared to placebo in the total number of asthma attacks that required treatment with corticosteroids or unscheduled medical visits. There was a reduction in beta-agonist use in both montelukast groups compared to placebo.[39]

The PREvention of Virally Induced Asthma trial was a multicenter, double-blind, parallel-group study of 549 children aged 2 to 5 years with a history of intermittent asthma symptoms.[40] Children were randomized to either daily montelukast or placebo for the 12 month treatment period. In children treated with montelukast, the average yearly asthma exacerbation rate was significantly lower than that of the placebo group by

31.8%. In addition, montelukast extended the time to the first exacerbation by 2 months and lowered the rate of inhaled corticosteroid use.

The Acute Intermittent Management Strategies (AIMS) trial was a randomized, double-blind, placebo-controlled study evaluating 238 children aged 12 to 59 months with a history of at least 2 wheezing respiratory tract infections in the preceding year with one episode within the last 6 months.[41] There were 3 treatment groups consisting of montelukast, ICS, and placebo with all treatment arms including albuterol as needed for the 12 months study period. There was no significant difference in episode-free days, OCS use, health-care use, linear growth, or quality of life among the 3 treatment groups. In participants with a positive mAPI, both montelukast and ICS improved breathing scores, interference with activity scores, and total symptom scores compared with placebo. For those with a negative mAPI, the study showed improvement only in the interference with activity score in the cohort receiving montelukast. Similar to the INFANT trial, 25% of children with asthma responded best to LTRA, though mAPI did not determine which treatment (daily ICS, intermittent PRN, or LTRA) the children would respond to best.[32]

A Cochrane meta-analysis was performed on 5 studies evaluating LTRAs as maintenance and intermittent therapy for episodic wheezing in children aged 1 to 6 years.[42] Although individual studies did show some benefit of LTRA therapy, the authors determined that there was no evidence of benefit from maintenance or intermittent LTRA treatment compared with placebo in decreasing the number of viral-induced wheezing episodes requiring rescue OCS.

The Wheeze And Intermittent Treatment study was a multicenter, randomized, placebo-controlled, parallel-group study to assess the efficacy of intermittent montelukast.[43] Enrollment included 1358 children aged 10 months to 5 years with a history of 2 or more wheezing episodes, 1 in the preceding 3 months. Children were allowed to continue their baseline medications that could include bronchodilators and ICS. Montelukast or placebo was started at home at the onset of wheezing or viral infection for more than a 12-month period. The intermittent montelukast cohort required fewer courses of OCS. No differences were seen in the number of wheezing episodes, duration of wheezing episodes, or unscheduled medical visits. In 2004 and updated in 2020, the US Food and Drug Administration added a black box label to montelukast stating that serious mental health side effects may include suicidal thoughts or actions have been reported in patients.[44]

Oral Corticosteroids

OCS are a mainstay of treatment of asthma exacerbation; however, in preschool children, OCS have not been consistently shown to be beneficial in wheezing episodes.[45,46] This may be due to the fact that many preschool children who wheeze do not develop asthma. One of the earlier studies looking at hospital admission rates recruited 74 participants aged 7 to 54 months who were evaluated in the ED for acute wheezing.[47] In this double-blind trial, participants received either a dose of intramuscular methylprednisone or placebo.[47] Patients were evaluated 3 hours after treatment with 20% of the methlyprednisone cohort being admitted to the hospital compared with 43% of the placebo cohort. This was more significant in children aged 7 to 24 months with only 18% of the treatment group requiring admission compared with 50% of the placebo group. The older children aged 24 to 54 months had a smaller difference in admission rates with 23% versus 31% requiring admission.[47]

Another study involving 230 children aged 6 to 35 months presenting to the ED with acute respiratory distress were randomized to 3 days of oral prednisone versus placebo.[48] Children were hospitalized at similar rates between the 2 groups but those treated with OCS had a shorter hospital duration by 1 day, 2 versus 3 days, in treatment versus placebo cohorts, respectively. Additionally, when compared with the placebo cohort, the treatment group had decreased need for additional asthma medication and shorter duration of symptoms by 1 day compared with the placebo group.

An Australian ED randomized, double-blind, placebo-controlled trial evaluated 624 children aged 24 to 72 months presenting to the ED with virus-associated wheeze.[49] Participants were treated with oral prednisone for 3 days or placebo. The average length of stay was decreased in the treatment group at 370 minutes compared with 540 minutes in the placebo group. This study found that in children with more severe symptoms, children who used albuterol before ED presentation and previously diagnosed with asthma were more likely to improve with OCS use. Another ED study treated 687 infants aged 10 to 60 months without bronchiolitis who presented to the ED with acute viral wheezing.[50] In this double-blind, placebo controlled study, children were randomized to prednisolone for 5 days versus placebo. There was no significant difference noted in the duration of hospitalization, albuterol use, or 7-day symptom score.

Seventy-nine children aged 3 to 23 months were evaluated for the effects of OCS in rhinovirus wheeze.[51] Children with an initial, acute, moderate–severe wheezing episode were randomized to receive 3 days of oral prednisone versus placebo and were followed for 12 months. Oral steroids improved short-term respiratory symptoms during the initial 2 weeks posttreatment. Long-term outcomes did not differ between treatment groups and included future wheezing episodes and controller medication for asthma. The use of home-administered OCS for viral-induced wheezing was evaluated in 108 children aged 1 to 5 years with a previous history of hospital admission for viral-induced wheeze.[52] These children were subsequently randomized to 5 days of OCS or placebo to use at that start of their next viral wheezing episode. There was no difference in daytime or nighttime lower respiratory tract symptoms, need for rescue medications, or hospital admission between the 2 groups or in children with above-average eosinophil priming determined by the level of serum eosinophil cationic protein greater than 20 mg/L and eosinophil protein X > 40 mg/L.

The following post hoc analysis focuses on OCS given for outpatient exacerbations in children who did not require ED evaluation. Beigelman and colleagues[53] performed a post hoc analysis on high-risk children enrolled in the AIMS trial and MIST trial; the investigators did not find any difference in total symptom score or length of symptoms during outpatient exacerbations among children who were treated or not treated with OCS. There were no risk factors that predicted which group of children would have greater benefit from OCS. Positive mAPI, atopic dermatitis, and family history of asthma are factors that would have been expected to yield greater benefit from OCS, although these groups did not have any additional benefit than those without atopic risk factors. Furthermore, there was also no difference noted in OCS treatment in patients on daily ICS versus no controller therapy as half of the children in the MIST trial were receiving daily ICS. This analysis shows minimal evidence to support the use of OCS in preschool children treated at home for intermittent viral wheezing.

The national and international asthma guidelines address OCS in young children with exacerbations. Updated asthma guidelines released by the Global Initiative for Asthma support consideration for OCS in children aged 5 years and younger if the child requires ED evaluation for hospital admission for exacerbation; OCS are not listed as a recommendation for outpatient exacerbation management.[54] The expert panel working group of the National Heart, Lung, and Blood Institute released an update to the national asthma management guidelines in 2020.[35] For children 4 years and younger with acute exacerbation, this group states to consider OCS if the child has a severe exacerbation or a history of severe exacerbations.[35] OCS can be beneficial in reducing hospital-based care in young children with a diagnosis of asthma, use of bronchodilators, and more severe wheezing episodes who seek ED evaluation; OCS are not in the list of recommendations for outpatient exacerbation management.[49] Additional studies are still needed in young children to best determine which subgroups will receive the greatest benefit from OCS.

Azithromycin

Bacteria, specifically S. pneumoniae and M. catarrhalis, are often detected in children who wheeze, both with and without the presence of viral infections.[18] As such, azithromycin has been studied in wheezing children. In the Copenhagen Prospective Study on Asthma in Childhood 2000 birth cohort, 72 children aged 1 to 3 years with a history of recurrent asthma symptoms were enrolled in a study to assess the duration of wheezing episodes when treated with azithromycin.[55] Children were randomized to receive 3 days of azithromycin or placebo with each wheezing episode of 3 consecutive days in duration. Azithromycin shortened the duration of symptoms to 3.4 days comparted to 7.7 with placebo, corresponding to a calculated reduction in episode length of 63.3%. Greater improvement was seen when the treatment was started earlier in the episode; however, treatment did not significantly affect the time to next episode of respiratory symptoms.

The Azithromycin for Preventing the Development of Upper Respiratory Tract Illness into Lower Respiratory Tract Symptoms in Children study was a randomized, double-blind, placebo-controlled, parallel-group trial evaluating intermittent azithromycin for respiratory tract infections.[56] Participants included 607 children aged 12 to 71 months with a history of recurrent severe lower respiratory tract infections with minimal impairment between episodes. Children were treated with 5 days of azithromycin or placebo at the onset of respiratory tract illness before lower respiratory tract illness developed. A total of 937 respiratory tract infections were treated during a period of 12 to 18 months. Azithromycin significantly reduced the risk of progression to a severe lower respiratory tract infection by 37%. Antimicrobial resistance was evaluated in a subset of participates throughout the study. At initial randomization, azithromycin-resistant organisms were isolated from 5 of 41 treatment participants and 4 of 45 placebo participants. At the completion of the study, azithromycin-resistant organisms were identified in an additional 3 patients per group: 8 of 40 in the treatment cohort and 7 of 41 in the placebo cohort. As the placebo cohort had a similar rate of azithromycin resistance, this secondary outcome measure was not statistically significant. Further studies are needed to evaluate the potential increased risk in resistance.

The use of azithromycin in the prevention of future wheezing episodes has been looked at in this recent prospective, double-blind, placebo-controlled study of 200 children aged 1 to 18 months admitted with RSV bronchiolitis assigned to 14 days of azithromycin or placebo.[57] Despite evidence of biologic activity on nasal interleukin-8 levels, azithromycin did not reduce the risk of post-RSV recurrent wheeze during the 2 to 4 year observation period (47% in the azithromycin group vs 36% in the placebo group). There were no differences in the number of days with respiratory symptoms, annualized days with albuterol use, or number of subsequent antibiotic courses or OCS courses. A greater number of participants in the azithromycin group were given a diagnosis of asthma by the end of the trial data collection compared with placebo at 15.6% and 8.7%, respectively. The hazard ratio for having an asthma diagnosis by the end of data collection was 1.95. Although azithromycin is an option for treatment in intermittent wheezing children, it has not been effective for asthma

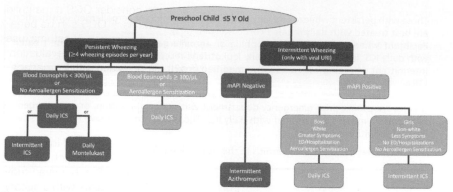

Fig. 1. Treatment Recommendations for Preschool Children with Wheeze. ICS, inhaled corticosteroid; mAPI, modified asthma predictive index.

prevention. **Fig. 1** illustrates the therapeutic options for the treatment of wheezing episodes in preschool children.

SUMMARY

Wheezing is common in childhood, although only a small percentage of these children develop asthma. The child's wheezing phenotype and asthma predictive indices help predict the likelihood of future asthma diagnosis. Lung function patterns are established in childhood where lung function deficits are established by 6 years of life. Viral infections are common in childhood with RSV accounting for most wheezing episodes in children aged less than 1 year and rhinovirus in children aged 1 year and greater. Many treatment options exist for wheezing children, including those that wheeze persistently or only due to viral infections. In atopic persistent wheezing children, daily ICS has been shown to be most effective. In nonatopic persistent wheezers, options include daily ICS, intermittent ICS, and daily montelukast. Intermittent wheezing children with a negative mAPI are best suited for intermittent azithromycin. Children intermittently wheezing with a positive mAPI and positive risk factors respond best to daily ICS, whereas those without risk factors can be treated with intermittent ICS. The benefit of OCS for exacerbations in this age is still inconclusive, although there is greater evidence to support OCS in those requiring ED evaluation or hospital admission.

CLINICS CARE POINTS

- Rhinovirus is the most common virus to cause wheezing in children aged 1 year and older. Wheezing with rhinovirus infection is a strong predictor of future wheezing episodes, and this prediction is higher in atopic individuals.

- Respiratory syncytial virus (RSV) is the most common virus to cause wheezing in children aged 1 year and younger. RSV lower respiratory tract illnesses before age 3 years is associated with a significant increase in risk of subsequent wheezing during the first 10 years but is not significant by age 13.

- The modified asthma predictive index and the pediatric asthma risk score are tools to identify infants at risk to develop asthma.

- Many treatment options are available for preschool children who wheeze:

- ○ Those with persistent wheeze and elevated blood eosinophils or aeroallergen sensitization are best treated with daily inhaled corticosteroids (ICS).
- ○ Persistent wheezing without eosinophilia or aeroallergen sensitization can be treated with daily ICS, intermittent ICS, or daily leukotriene receptor antagonist (LTRA).
- ○ Intermittent wheezing with a negative modified (mAPI) can be treated with intermittent LTRA.
- ○ Intermittent wheezing with a positive mAPI and risk factors of male gender, Caucasian, greater symptoms, prior emergency department visit or hospitalization, or aeroallergen sensitization may be best treated with daily ICS. Those without the above risk factors can be treated with intermittent ICS.

- The effectiveness of oral corticosteroids in this age range is inconclusive.

DISCLOSURES

A.M.A. Doss-nothing to disclose. J.R. Stokes: Research grants from NIH, Avillion LLP, Sanofi-Aventis/SA, and Regeneron Pharmaceuticals.

REFERENCES

1. Martinez FD, Wright AL, Taussig LM, et al. Asthma and wheezing in the first six years of life. N Engl J Med 1995;332(3):133–8.
2. Jackson DJ, Evans MD, Gangnon RE, et al. Evidence for a causal relationship between allergic sensitization and rhinovirus wheezing in early life. Am J Respir Crit Care Med 2012;185(3):281–5.
3. Johnson CC, Havstad SL, Ownby DR, et al. Pediatric asthma incidence rates in the United States from 1980 to 2017. J Allergy Clin Immunol 2021;148(5): 1270–80.
4. Pate CA, Zahran HS, Qin X, et al. Asthma Surveillance - United States, 2006-2018. MMWR Surveill Summ 2021;70(5):1–32.
5. Akinbami LJ, Moorman JE, Garbe PL, et al. Status of childhood asthma in the United States, 1980-2007. Pediatrics 2009;123(Suppl 3):S131–45.
6. Zahran HS, Bailey CM, Damon SA, et al. Vital signs: asthma in children - United States, 2001-2016. MMWR Morb Mortal Wkly Rep 2018;67(5):149–55.
7. Morgan WJ, Stern DA, Sherrill DL, et al. Outcome of asthma and wheezing in the first 6 years of life. Am J Respir Crit Care Med 2005;172(10):1253–8.
8. Savenije OE, Granell R, Caudri D, et al. Comparison of childhood wheezing phenotypes in 2 birth cohorts: ALSPAC and PIAMA. J Allergy Clin Immunol 2011; 127(6):1505–12.e14.
9. Oksel C, Granell R, Mahmoud O, et al. Causes of variability in latent phenotypes of childhood wheeze. J Allergy Clin Immunol 2019;143(5):1783–90.e11.
10. Henderson J, Granell R, Heron J, et al. Associations of wheezing phenotypes in the first 6 years of life with atopy, lung function and airway responsiveness in midchildhood. Thorax 2008;63(11):974–80.
11. Fitzpatrick AM, Bacharier LB, Guilbert TW, et al. Phenotypes of recurrent wheezing in preschool children: identification by latent class analysis and utility in prediction of future exacerbation. J Allergy Clin Immunol Pract 2019;7(3): 915–24.e7.
12. Bacharier LB, Beigelman A, Calatroni A, et al. Longitudinal phenotypes of respiratory health in a high-risk urban birth cohort. Am J Respir Crit Care Med 2019; 199(1):71–82.
13. Heikkinen T, Jarvinen A. The common cold. Lancet 2003;361(9351):51–9.

14. Rakes GP, Arruda E, Ingram JM, et al. Rhinovirus and respiratory syncytial virus in wheezing children requiring emergency care. Am J Respir Crit Care Med 1999; 159(3):785–90.

15. Johnston SL, Pattemore PK, Sanderson G, et al. Community study of role of viral infections in exacerbations of asthma in 9-11 year old children. BMJ 1995; 310(6989):1225–9.

16. Teo SM, Mok D, Pham K, et al. The infant nasopharyngeal microbiome impacts severity of lower respiratory infection and risk of asthma development. Cell Host Microbe 2015;17(5):704–15.

17. Lemanske RF Jr, Jackson DJ, Gangnon RE, et al. Rhinovirus illnesses during infancy predict subsequent childhood wheezing. J Allergy Clin Immunol 2005; 116(3):571–7.

18. Jackson DJ, Gern JE, Lemanske RF. The contributions of allergic sensitization and respiratory pathogens to asthma inception. J Allergy Clin Immunol 2016; 137(3):659–65.

19. Caliskan M, Bochkov YA, Kreiner-Moller E, et al. Rhinovirus wheezing illness and genetic risk of childhood-onset asthma. N Engl J Med 2013;368(15):1398–407.

20. Altman MC, Beigelman A, Ciaccio C, et al. Evolving concepts in how viruses impact asthma: a work group report of the microbes in allergy committee of the american academy of allergy, asthma & immunology. J Allergy Clin Immunol 2020;145(5):1332–44.

21. Stein RT, Sherrill D, Morgan WJ, et al. Respiratory syncytial virus in early life and risk of wheeze and allergy by age 13 years. Lancet 1999;354(9178):541–5.

22. Blanken MO, Rovers MM, Molenaar JM, et al. Respiratory syncytial virus and recurrent wheeze in healthy preterm infants. N Engl J Med 2013;368(19):1791–9.

23. Scheltema NM, Nibbelke EE, Pouw J, et al. Respiratory syncytial virus prevention and asthma in healthy preterm infants: a randomised controlled trial. Lancet Respir Med 2018;6(4):257–64.

24. Rubner FJ, Jackson DJ, Evans MD, et al. Early life rhinovirus wheezing, allergic sensitization, and asthma risk at adolescence. J Allergy Clin Immunol 2017; 139(2):501–7.

25. Carlsson CJ, Vissing NH, Sevelsted A, et al. Duration of wheezy episodes in early childhood is independent of the microbial trigger. J Allergy Clin Immunol 2015; 136(5):1208–14.e5.

26. Bisgaard H, Hermansen MN, Buchvald F, et al. Childhood asthma after bacterial colonization of the airway in neonates. N Engl J Med 2007;357(15):1487–95.

27. Kloepfer KM, Lee WM, Pappas TE, et al. Detection of pathogenic bacteria during rhinovirus infection is associated with increased respiratory symptoms and asthma exacerbations. J Allergy Clin Immunol 2014;133(5):1301–7.e3.

28. Castro-Rodríguez JA, Holberg CJ, Wright AL, et al. A clinical index to define risk of asthma in young children with recurrent wheezing. Am J Respir Crit Care Med 2000;162(4):1403–6.

29. Guilbert TW, Morgan WJ, Krawiec M, et al. The prevention of early asthma in kids study: design, rationale and methods for the childhood asthma research and education network. Controlled Clin Trials 2004;25(3):286–310.

30. Chang TS, Lemanske RF, Guilbert TW, et al. Evaluation of the modified asthma predictive index in high-risk preschool children. J Allergy Clin Immunol Pract 2013;1(2):152–6.

31. Biagini Myers JM, Schauberger E, He H, et al. A pediatric asthma risk score to better predict asthma development in young children. J Allergy Clin Immunol 2019;143(5):1803–10.e2.

32. Fitzpatrick AM, Jackson DJ, Mauger DT, et al. Individualized therapy for persistent asthma in young children. J Allergy Clin Immunol 2016;138(6):1608–18.e12.
33. Papi A, Nicolini G, Baraldi E, et al. Regular vs prn nebulized treatment in wheeze preschool children. Allergy 2009;64(10):1463–71.
34. Kaiser SV, Huynh T, Bacharier LB, et al. Preventing exacerbations in preschoolers with recurrent wheeze: a meta-analysis. Pediatrics 2016;137(6):e20154496.
35. Cloutier MM, Baptist AP, Blake KV, et al. 2020 Focused updates to the asthma management guidelines: a report from the national asthma education and prevention program coordinating committee expert panel working group. J Allergy Clin Immunol 2020;146(6):1217–70.
36. Zeiger RS, Mauger D, Bacharier LB, et al. Daily or intermittent budesonide in preschool children with recurrent wheezing. N Engl J Med 2011;365(21):1990–2001.
37. Bisgaard H, Hermansen MN, Loland L, et al. Intermittent inhaled corticosteroids in infants with episodic wheezing. N Engl J Med 2006;354(19):1998–2005.
38. Ducharme FM, Lemire C, Noya FJD, et al. Preemptive use of high-dose fluticasone for virus-induced wheezing in young children. N Engl J Med 2009;360(4):339–53.
39. Valovirta E, Boza ML, Robertson CF, et al. Intermittent or daily montelukast versus placebo for episodic asthma in children. Ann Allergy Asthma Immunol 2011;106(6):518–26.
40. Bisgaard H, Zielen S, Garcia-Garcia ML, et al. Montelukast Reduces Asthma Exacerbations in 2- to 5-Year-Old Children with Intermittent Asthma. Am J Respir Crit Care Med 2005;171(4):315–22.
41. Bacharier LB, Phillips BR, Zeiger RS, et al. Episodic use of an inhaled corticosteroid or leukotriene receptor antagonist in preschool children with moderate-to-severe intermittent wheezing. J Allergy Clin Immunol 2008;122(6):1127–35.e8.
42. Brodlie M, Gupta A, Rodriguez-Martinez CE, et al. Leukotriene receptor antagonists as maintenance and intermittent therapy for episodic viral wheeze in children. Cochrane Database Syst Rev 2015;2020(1):CD008202.
43. Nwokoro C, Pandya H, Turner S, et al. Intermittent montelukast in children aged 10 months to 5 years with wheeze (WAIT trial): a multicentre, randomised, placebo-controlled trial. Lancet Respir Med 2014;2(10):796–803.
44. Clarridge K, Chin S, Eworuke E, et al. A boxed warning for montelukast: the FDA perspective. J Allergy Clin Immunol Pract 2021;9(7):2638–41.
45. Beigelman A, Durrani S, Guilbert TW. Should a preschool child with acute episodic wheeze be treated with oral corticosteroids? A Pro/Con Debate. J Allergy Clin Immunol Pract 2016;4(1):27–35.
46. Stokes JR, Bacharier LB. Prevention and treatment of recurrent viral-induced wheezing in the preschool child. Ann Allergy Asthma Immunol 2020;125(2):156–62.
47. Tal A, Levy N, Bearman JE. Methylprednisolone therapy for acute asthma in infants and toddlers: a controlled clinical trial. Pediatrics 1990;86(3):350–6.
48. Csonka P, Kaila M, Laippala P, et al. Oral prednisolone in the acute management of children age 6 to 35 months with viral respiratory infection-induced lower airway disease: a randomized, placebo-controlled trial. J Pediatr 2003;143(6):725–30.
49. Foster SJ, Cooper MN, Oosterhof S, et al. Oral prednisolone in preschool children with virus-associated wheeze: a prospective, randomised, double-blind, placebo-controlled trial. Lancet Respir Med 2018;6(2):97–106.
50. Panickar J, Lakhanpaul M, Lambert PC, et al. Oral prednisolone for preschool children with acute virus-induced wheezing. N Engl J Med 2009;360(4):329–38.

51. Jartti T, Nieminen R, Vuorinen T, et al. Short- and long-term efficacy of predniso-lone for first acute rhinovirus-induced wheezing episode. J Allergy Clin Immunol 2015;135(3):691–698 e9.

52. Oommen A, Lambert PC, Grigg J. Efficacy of a short course of parent-initiated oral prednisolone for viral wheeze in children aged 1–5 years: randomised controlled trial. Lancet 2003;362(9394):1433–8.

53. Beigelman A, King TS, Mauger D, et al. Do oral corticosteroids reduce the severity of acute lower respiratory tract illnesses in preschool children with recur-rent wheezing? J Allergy Clin Immunol 2013;131(6):1518–25.

54. Reddel HK, Bacharier LB, Bateman ED, et al. Global initiative for asthma strategy 2021. executive summary and rationale for key changes. Arch Bronconeumol 2022;58(1):35–51.

55. Stokholm J, Chawes BL, Vissing NH, et al. Azithromycin for episodes with asthma-like symptoms in young children aged 1–3 years: a randomised, double-blind, placebo-controlled trial. Lancet Respir Med 2016;4(1):19–26.

56. Bacharier LB, Guilbert TW, Mauger DT, et al. Early administration of azithromycin and prevention of severe lower respiratory tract illnesses in preschool children with a history of such illnesses. JAMA 2015;314(19):2034.

57. Beigelman A, Srinivasan M, Goss CW, et al. Azithromycin to prevent recurrent wheeze following severe respiratory syncytial virus bronchiolitis. NEJM Evid 2022;1(4). https://doi.org/10.1056/EVIDoa2100069.

Environmental Exposures Impact Pediatric Asthma Within the School Environment

Caroline L. Mortelliti, MS[a], Tina M. Banzon, MD[a],
Carolina Zilli Vieira, PhD, DDS[b], Wanda Phipatanakul, MD, MS[a],*

KEYWORDS

- School inner-city asthma study (SICAS) • Pediatrics • Indoor allergens
- Allergen exposure • Childhood asthma • School-based interventions
- Integrated pest management • HEPA filter

KEY POINTS

- Children with asthma suffer from increased asthma morbidity following exposure to common school-based biologic allergens such as cockroach, mouse, cat and dog, classroom pets, dust mite, fungus, and mold.
- Children with asthma experience increased asthma morbidity following exposure to school-based air pollutants in the physical environment, including particulate matter (PM), carbon monoxide (CO), nitrogen dioxide (NO_2), black carbon (BC), and sulfur dioxide (SO_2).
- Asthma prevalence and asthma-associated health care needs are exacerbated among inner-city children in areas with high levels of poverty and large minority populations.
- School-based interventions to reduce classroom exposures have had mixed outcomes. Ongoing research is needed to determine the effectiveness of these interventions in improving the health of those attending schools.

INTRODUCTION

Asthma is one of the leading chronic medical conditions in the United States, affecting more than 24 million people.[1] Of those, approximately 5.8%, or 6 million individuals, are children less than the age of 18 years.[1,2] Early life aeroallergen sensitization increases a child's risk of developing adolescent asthma, with Rubner and colleagues[3] demonstrating that children who were sensitized to aeroallergens during early life (age 1–5 years) were more likely to develop asthma. In this study, 65% of children

[a] Boston Children's Hospital, 300 Longwood Avenue, Fegan 6, Boston, MA 02115, USA; [b] EH - Exposure Epidemiology and Risk Program, Harvard TH Chan School of Public Health, Landmark Center West, Room 420401 Park Dr, Boston, MA 02215, USA
* Corresponding author.
E-mail address: Wanda.Phipatanakul@childrens.harvard.edu

Immunol Allergy Clin N Am 42 (2022) 743–760
https://doi.org/10.1016/j.iac.2022.05.005
0889-8561/22/© 2022 Elsevier Inc. All rights reserved.

sensitized by age 1% and 40% of children sensitized by age 5 developed persistent asthma by age 13.[3] A causative relationship between early childhood exposure and asthma development remains under active study; though, early life aeroallergen sensitization may be helpful to identify a cohort of children predisposed to asthma.

A national US study showed individuals will spend an average of 87% of their time indoors, and about 6% of their time in vehicles.[4] Toddlers and children spend an estimated 7 to 12 hours per day in daycare or in school buildings. Given the majority of individuals will spend most of their time indoors, the indoor environment has been investigated for environmental exposures that might predispose occupants to asthma. Initial home investigations found that most inner-city children with moderate to severe asthma are sensitized to multiple indoor home allergens (cockroach, rodents, cat/dog dander, tobacco smoke, and dust mites), with these environmental allergens known to be associated with asthma severity and asthma morbidity.[5,6] Studies have since expanded beyond the home to understand environmental exposures in the school setting. These investigations demonstrated a strong association between school environmental exposures and childhood asthma morbidity.[7-11] Thus, the school environment is now recognized as an important contributor to childhood asthma. Air pollutants and irritants in the physical environment in both the home and school also contribute to asthma morbidity and will be discussed.

To date, there is no cure for asthma disease. Prevention strategies are aimed at attenuating IgE antibody production and mitigating downstream inflammatory processes.[3,12] This review will focus on common allergens as well as physical exposures in the school setting, and the impact of these environmental exposures on children with asthma. Additionally, school-based intervention strategies intended to reduce asthma morbidity will be reviewed. Understanding influential factors in the environments of children with asthma are integral to the management and improvement of current and future asthma diseases. Additionally, asthma prevalence and health care needs associated with asthma are often exacerbated by socioeconomic and minority status,[6] prompting a need to better understand asthma development and its association with environmental allergen exposure as it relates to health care disparities.

BIOLOGIC ALLERGENS
Cockroach

Cockroach is highly prevalent within crowded urban homes of low-income families.[13] Sensitization to cockroach was reported in 60%–80% of inner-city children living with asthma, and in only 21% of suburban children with asthma.[13] The major cockroach allergens responsible for cockroach associated morbidity are Bla g 1 and Bla g 2, though recently, the number of relevant cockroach allergens has expanded to 12 groups.[14] The National Cooperative Inner-City Asthma Study (NCICAS) reported that cockroach exposure in inner-city homes is significantly linked to asthma exacerbation and higher asthma morbidity.[5,6] Children experience longer asthma symptom days, missed school days, loss of sleep, asthma-related hospitalizations, and unscheduled medical visits.[5] Additionally, studies indicate that increased cockroach exposures greater than 1 U/g lead to cockroach sensitization.[15,16]

From a school and classroom perspective, the most effective intervention for cockroach elimination involves professional integrated pest management (IPM), which can reduce exposure by up to 90%.[17] Otherwise, mitigation strategies include removal of food sources, blocking mechanisms of entry, and eliminating cockroaches already present in the area through traps and insecticide.[18] However, these interventions have yielded mixed results. The Inner-City Asthma Study (ICAS) demonstrated that a home-based "multifaceted" intervention (removal of more than one asthma trigger at once) effectively decreased cockroach exposure, and improved asthma symptoms for a year after the intervention ended.[19] Meanwhile, DiMango and colleagues[20] performed another multifaceted intervention that significantly reduced the amount of allergen in New York City homes, but did not reduce the use of asthma controller therapy (**Table 1**). Alternatively, Rabito and colleagues[17] performed a single intervention against cockroach using insecticidal bait which was successful in reducing cockroach number and cockroach allergen improving asthma outcomes (see **Table 1**).

Addressing school-based interventions, the School Inner-City Asthma intervention study (SICAS-2) aimed to reduce school-specific exposures. More than 90% of baseline classroom cockroach levels were undetectable, and so efforts were focused more on mouse allergen.[21] To date, there has still not been a successful intervention to reduce the number of cockroach allergen or live cockroach in the school setting. However, the use of insecticidal bait following the methodology of Rabito and colleagues may provide a hopeful approach.

Mouse

Mouse allergen exposure is also associated with increased childhood asthma morbidity.[22–24] Mouse allergenic proteins Mus m 1 and Mus m 2 are found in mouse urine, dander, and hair follicles.[12] These mouse proteins are ubiquitous in the indoor environment, and are present in suburban and urban homes, and especially in schools.[25] In 2004, a US national survey reported that 82% of family homes had detectable amounts of mouse allergen.[26] Later, through the NCICAS study, Phipatanakul and colleagues showed that subjects whose homes had increased mouse allergen concentrations had increased rates of mouse sensitization.[24]

In 2021, a survey of a northeastern US city reported that 98% of its inner-city classrooms had detectable mouse allergen.[21] A subsequent study by Sheehan and colleagues[8] indicated that levels of mouse allergen in these same classrooms were higher than levels of mouse allergen in students' homes, indicating that the classroom should be a site of increased pest management efforts. Sheehan and colleagues[8] also importantly revealed that school mouse allergen is associated with increased asthma symptoms and worsened pulmonary function in children, independent of allergen sensitization status.

In 2017, the Mouse Allergen and Asthma Intervention Trial (MAAIT) randomized mouse sensitized children with asthma to receive long-term home IPM with pest management education, or pest management education alone (see **Table 1**). Home IPM strategies included (1) identifying pest population locations with sticky traps, (2) blocking entry ways, (3) removing possible sources of food/water, and (4) terminating pest count with low-toxicity pesticides. Mouse allergen levels decreased substantially in both groups (approximately 70% reduction).[27] While there was no significant reduction in asthma symptom days between the 2 groups, there was an association between greater reduction in mouse allergen and more improved clinical benefit.[27] In post hoc analysis, homes in which either arm had 90% reductions in mouse allergen exposure had clinical benefits similar to effects seen with inhaled corticosteroids in the childhood asthma management program (CAMP).[27–29] Additionally, the intervention may have implications for long-term health benefits, as children who experienced a 75% reduction in mouse allergen exposure had significantly increased projection in lung growth.[27]

In an effort to study the effects of mouse allergen in the school, the NIH/NIAID-funded School Inner City Asthma Study (SICAS-1; adjusted for home exposures) revealed that exposure to classroom mouse allergen did, in fact, increase asthma

Table 1
Select intervention study results evaluating reduction in aeroallergen exposure and health outcomes (2001–2021)

Reference (y)	Allergens Targeted	Population	Intervention	Trial Results: Allergen Outcomes	Trial Results: Health Outcomes
Carter et al,[55] 2001	DM, cockroach	104 inner-city-individuals with asthma aged 6–16 y	Intervention group received allergen-impermeable covers, cockroach bait, education regarding DM and roach limitation. Placebo group received (sham) allergen-permeable covers, instructions to wash in cold water. Control group received medical care	Substantial reduction defined as a 70% decrease, no difference found between intervention and placebo groups	Reduction in acute visits for asthma in intervention group Decreased acute visits in those with DM allergy who had decreased DM exposure
Morgan et al,[10] 2004	Indoor allergens and tobacco smoke	937 inner-city individuals with asthma and aeroallergen sensitization aged 5–11 y	Intervention group received 1 y of education, allergen-impermeable covers, HEPA vacuum and bedroom filter, personalized education, and IPM based on sensitization and exposure Control group evaluation every 6 mo	Reduced DM, cockroach allergen levels	Reduction in urgent visits Decreased asthma symptom days during the intervention year and the following year
Eggleston et al,[56] 2005	Indoor allergens (cockroach, mouse) PM_{10} and $PM_{2.5}$	100 low-income 6- to 12-y-old individuals with asthma	Intervention group 1 y of education, allergen-impermeable covers, bedroom HEPA filter, IPM based on sensitization and exposure Control group treatment at end of 1 y	Approx. 50% reduction in cockroach allergen level, approx. 39% reduction in PM_{10} and $PM_{2.5}$	Reduction in daytime asthma symptoms

Bryant Stephens et al,[57] 2009	DM, pests, pets, tobacco smoke	264 individuals with asthma aged 2–16 y	Two intervention groups, 1 immediate and 1 delayed: education, allergen-impermeable covers, cockroach bait, mice traps, replacement carpet, curtains	Reductions were seen in pests, presence of carpets in bedrooms, and dust.	Nighttime wheezing significantly reduced after the intervention in both groups (P < .001). Mean number of emergency visits decreased by 30% after the intervention. Inpatient visits decrease by 54% (P < .001) after the intervention.
DiMango et al,[44] 2016	DM, cockroach, mouse, cat, dog	110 adults with asthma and 137 children with asthma, all with aeroallergen sensitization	Asthma control optimized before randomization. Intervention group 40-wk education, allergen-impermeable covers, bedroom HEPA filter, and HEPA vacuum Control group education not including allergen avoidance	Intervention group displayed reduced DM, cockroach, mouse, cat, dog Control group: reduced cockroach, DM, and mouse	Asthma control improved in both groups
Matsui et al,[35] 2017	Mouse allergen	350 children with asthma who were sensitized and exposed to mouse allergen	Intervention group Rodenticide, sealing portals of rodent entry, traps, allergen-impermeable covers, HEPA filter. If mice remained, further treatment to eliminate infestation Control group education regarding mechanisms	Approximately 70% reduction in mouse allergen in both groups, no difference in allergen levels between them	Reduction in mouse allergen associated with improvements in asthma symptoms, rescue inhaler use, urgent visits. No difference in symptoms between groups.

(continued on next page)

Table 1
(continued)

Reference (y)	Allergens Targeted	Population	Intervention	Trial Results: Allergen Outcomes	Trial Results: Health Outcomes
Rabito et al,[43] 2017	Cockroach allergen	102 individuals with moderate-severe asthma aged 5-7 y, homes cockroach-infested	Intervention group cockroach trapping and baiting at 0, 1, 3, 6, 9, and 12 mo Control group cockroach trapping, but no baiting, at 0, 1, 3, 6, 9, and 12 mo	Reduction in cockroach in homes with trapping and baiting	Reduced asthma symptoms and urgent health visits Less participants with FEV1 < 80% predicted
Murray et al,[11] 2017	DM allergen	286 DM- sensitized individuals with prior emergency hospital visits	Intervention group 12 mo with allergen-impermeable covers for bed Control group 12 mo with no allergen-impermeable covers	Mattres DM level reduced by 84% in the intervention group, no change in the placebo group ($P < .001$). Floor DM levels unchanged in both groups ($P = .48$).	Reduction in hospital visits for asthma exacerbation. No reduction in need for oral corticosteroids.
Phipatanakul et al,[31] 2021	Mouse, rat, cat, dog, DM, mold, allergens	236 elementary students with asthma	Intervention group school-wide IPM (rodenticide, sealing entry, traps, cleaning, education). Additional treatments for infestation. Classroom HEPA filters. Control group No IPM, sham classroom HEPA filters	At baseline, 98% of classrooms had detectable mouse allergen. More than 90% of baseline levels for cockroach, rat, Alternaria, Aspergillus, DM were undetectable. IPM dis not significantly reduce any measured allergens. HEPA filters significantly reduced airborne mouse and dog allergen	Asthma symptom days decreased by 0.4 d in the schools with IPM. After the use of HEPA filters in classrooms, asthma symptom days were reduced by 0.2. Neither produced a significant reduction in asthma symptom days overall. Post hoc, IPM reduced asthma symptoms significantly by 63% early in the school year during the fall and winter exacerbation season, but the benefit was not sustained

From Maciag MC, Phipatanakul W. Update on indoor allergens and their impact on pediatric asthma [published online ahead of print, 2022 Feb 25]. Ann Allergy Asthma Immunol. 2022:S1081-1206(22)00119-3.

symptoms and decreased lung function.[8,30] The SICAS-2 intervention, which was a school-wide IPM strategy and a classroom high-efficiency particulate air (HEPA) filter strategy, identified that IPM reduced asthma symptoms by 63% in the fall and winter seasons compared with control; however, this effect was not sustained.[21] Secondarily, IPM did reduce school days missed due to asthma.[21] Interestingly, classroom HEPA filters, while reducing particles and exposures, did not improve health outcomes or reduced asthma symptoms (see **Table 1**). Further study is necessary to determine what strategies could help sustain benefit and may need an approach targeting more susceptible children with certain baseline levels of exposure, which SICAS-2 was not practically designed to test.[21,31]

Cat and Dog

Previous studies demonstrate that levels of cat and dog exposure are associated with allergen sensitization and asthma symptoms.[32,33] An estimated 68% of households (84.6 million homes) in the United States own a pet.[34] Therefore, there is significant in-home exposure and sensitization to animals. However, animal exposure extends far beyond the house.[32,33] Cat and dog allergens (Fel d 1 and Can f 1, respectively) are carried on airborne particles and can be distributed between humans by textiles and carpeting, clothing, and human hair.[35,36] A recent study shows most teenagers allergic to cats were not cat owners themselves.[37] This raises questions about the ability by which individuals can be sensitized outside their homes.

Schools and daycares have been identified as high-risk sites for cat and dog allergen exposure, as children spend anywhere from 7 to 12 hours a day in these environments. Many studies have found that cat and dog allergen levels in schools far exceed the threshold of sensitization,[32,33,38,39] and that schools have more cat and dog allergen than do households without pets.[38–40] The case for hypoallergenic dogs remains unsubstantiated, as Can f 1 levels are similar between hypoallergenic breeds, and those that are not.[41] However, levels of these allergens are subject to change between schools and are dependent on a number of factors. The number of pet owners in a classroom is one of the strongest predictors of cat or dog allergen,[11,38] as well as the presence of carpeted floors and fabric materials. The latter are of more concern for elementary and preschool children during play, especially as this exposure may come during a period of early life sensitization susceptibility.[3]

Previously published SICAS studies demonstrate that dog and cat allergens were frequently detected in schools; however, these levels were found to be below the threshold levels associated with asthma symptoms.[8,15,42] Possible explanations for these relatively low dog and cat allergens might be due to an overall lower prevalence of household pet ownership in inner-city communities, introducing fewer allergens into schools.[8]

A potential mitigation strategy for reducing the level of pet allergen in the home, school, or other communities, is to modify cats' diet using anti-Fel d 1 immunoglobulin Y. Ingestion of this neutralizing antibody is associated with a reduction in allergen levels and improvement of owner's allergic rhinitis, and potentially asthma symptoms.[16] Perhaps of more universal use to homes and schools in the use of HEPA filters, HEPA integrated vacuums, and frequent washing of pets.[41] The SICAS-2 intervention study demonstrates that use of HEPA filters significantly reduced airborne mouse and dog allergens in classrooms.[21]

Classroom Pets (Guinea Pigs, Hamsters, Rabbits)

Many classrooms throughout the US have class pets. In a previous survey, it was reported that about 25% of sampled elementary school teachers endorsed having a classroom animal, mostly a small vertebrate.[43] In 2015, the American Humane Association determined that the most common classroom pets were fish (31%), guinea pigs (13.7%), and hamsters (10.5%).[44] To date, there are no studies assessing the environmental risk of these pets, their effects on sensitization, atopic disease, or asthma morbidity. Investigation into this impactful niche is available for future study.

Dust Mite

Dust mites (DM) are a major ubiquitous environmental allergen.[18] The two most common DM species found in the US are *Dermatophagoides farinae* (Der f 1) and *Dermatophagoides pteronyssinus* (Der p 1).[18] DM thrive in warm environments with humidity greater than 50%[45] and flourish in bedding, carpeting, upholstery, older single-family homes, and homes without air conditioning–which keep the humidity high and dust sources undisturbed.[18,45] Demographic factors also play a role in increasing DM exposure: higher population density, lower income households, and coexistence of DM with cockroach and mold all increase human exposure.[46] Previous studies have demonstrated an association between DM allergen exposure and sensitization, whereby exposure of greater than 2 ug/g results in mite sensitization.[47] Similarly, the threshold level of DM exposure associated with asthma symptom onset is > 10 ug/g (equivalent to 500 mites/g dust), with studies reporting DM allergen exposure to be associated with asthma exacerbation in children sensitized to DM.[46,48]

Within the school setting, DM levels vary largely depending on classroom features. DM are higher in carpeted classrooms, which are often reserved for play in elementary and preschools.[49] DM is high during the playtime hour itself, when activity across the carpet disrupts allergens making them airborne.[50] While DM allergen levels in schools and daycares have been found to far exceed sensitization thresholds (>2 ug/g), the mean and/or median DM concentrations are still below the asthma symptom threshold (>10 ug/g).[15,38,42,46,48]

In terms of DM mitigation, many home strategies might be transferable to the classroom such as total removal of extraneous fabrics and upholstery or washing of fabrics and upholstery using hot water once a week.[51,52] HEPA room filters can also trap particles as small as 0.1 mm, but may disturb DM on the floor.[53] Some DM reduction trials have successfully reduced DM levels and complications of asthma.[19] A 2017 home-study by Murray and colleagues[54] demonstrated that use of allergen-impermeable bed covers reduced mattress dust mite levels by 84% and reduced hospital visits for asthma exacerbation, but did not lessen the need for medication (see **Table 1**). The SICAS-2 intervention assessed airborne and settled DM exposure effects on asthma outcomes, but more than 90% of baseline classroom DM levels were undetectable, and were not used in further analysis (see **Table 1**).[21] Across multiple studies, management of sustained DM reduction and associated improved health outcomes remains ongoing.

Fungus and Mold

Fungi are ubiquitous organisms present in outdoor and indoor environments. Airborne fungal spores enter indoor environments through open windows and doors and accumulate on indoor surfaces. When inhaled, fungal spores are thought to cause adverse health effects, especially in those who are sensitized to mold or have underlying respiratory diseases. The threshold level of fungal exposure that is associated with asthma onset is not yet known, but it is expected that each fungal species impacts asthma onset in a different manner with a unique threshold. Overall, several studies have determined that there is a significant association between indoor fungus and asthma symptoms.[46,55–59]

Multiple studies have demonstrated that schools and classrooms are susceptible to fungus exposure and that fungus exposure has implications for allergic disease. In a SICAS study, Baxi and colleagues[60] demonstrated that in schools located in the northeastern United States, exposure to *Alternaria* was significantly associated with asthma symptom days in a dose-dependent manner among students already sensitized to *Alternaria*. Studies from other countries have found similar results. Simoni and colleagues[61] identified an association between *Aspergillus* and *Penicillium* fungal exposure in the classroom with asthma morbidity and night coughs. In Taiwan, Chen and colleagues[9] demonstrated that classroom *Aspergillus* and *Penicillium* spore exposure was associated with asthma and that asthma symptoms were reduced when children stayed home for holiday. In Portugal, investigators interestingly found that exposure to greater fungal diversity was protective against allergic sensitization to all fungus and indoor molds, but was not protective against asthma.[62]

Tactics for reducing indoor fungal exposure can be used in both the home and school environments: eliminating moisture, applying fungicides, and removing contaminated materials. However, interventions have had mixed asthma outcomes.[63,64] There are several considerations as to why fungal interventions have had variable success. In general, fungal exposure to health is understudied and unpredictable. Diversity of molds and fungus in the environment and the timing of their exposure may alter pulmonary health outcomes in numerous ways.[65] There is thoughtful consideration to continue intervention studies in the school environment, rather than the individualized home, as the former has the potential to impact many students simultaneously and potentially make larger clinical advancements.

Molds are a type of fungus with exposures linked to asthma development and exacerbation.[66,67] The Environmental Relative Moldiness Index (ERMI) has been successfully used to predict the asthma-related health effects of mold exposures in homes.[66,67] A SICAS analysis by Howard and colleagues[66] assessed the difference between ERMI values in homes and schools in the northeast US and found that levels of outdoor-sourced group 2 molds were significantly higher in schools. Simultaneously, the presence of school air conditioning significantly correlated with lower asthma prevalence. Together, these findings suggest that interventions such as SICAS-2 or other methods to improve air quality may be helpful in reducing asthma symptoms.[66]

The SICAS-2 intervention aimed to investigate fungi in the school environment; however, levels of common fungi *Alternaria* and *Aspergillus* were undetectable at baseline (see **Table 1**).[21] Although HEPA filters overall did not improve health outcomes in SICAS-2, in a subset of children with high mold exposure, HEPA filters were effective.[21,68] In post hoc analysis, HEPA filtration interventions on mold levels were quantified using ERMI, and possible improvement of asthma symptoms was quantified with spirometry testing. Classroom HEPA interventions significantly reduced ERMI values which corresponded to significant improvements in the students' FEV_1 outcomes, when compared with control sham filters.[68]

Microbiome

The microbiome is the combination of all microbes colonizing skin and mucosal surfaces. Microbial imbalance within the human body has been linked to altered risk of asthma development later in life.[69] However, recent data from Lai and colleagues[70] suggest that external microbiomes may contribute to the development and/or exacerbation of asthma symptoms. This study found that the composition of the home and school microbiomes significantly differed, and that classroom microbial diversity was associated with significantly increased asthma symptom days. Additionally, the classroom microbiome is modifiable by IPM but not HEPA filtration.[70]

PHYSICAL ENVIRONMENT
Air Pollution

Exposure to air pollution has been associated with long-term health effects including worsening of asthma symptoms, decreased lung function, increased medication use, hospital visits, and overall mortality.[71–74] Air pollution is a ubiquitous combination of airborne pollutants, including particulate matter (PM), carbon monoxide (CO), nitrogen dioxide (NO_2), black carbon (BC), and sulfur dioxide (SO_2).[75] PM is composed of airborne particles, including $PM_{2.5}$, $PM_{2.5-10}$ or PM_{10} (aerodynamic diameter of 2.5–10 microns).[76,77] $PM_{2.5}$ is associated with worsening asthma symptoms and increased oxidative stress based on elevated inflammatory biomarkers.[76] Overall, there is less data on the long-term health consequences of $PM_{2.5-10}$ because of the lack of monitoring locations of each pollutant. It is generally thought that $PM_{2.5-10}$ is less harmful than $PM_{2.5}$ due to its larger size and diminished lung penetration, but even still, $PM_{2.5-10}$ is associated with increased asthma diagnosis prevalence and health care utilization.[78]

There is strong evidence to suggest that ambient air pollution can exacerbate preexisting asthma. Exposure to NO_2, $PM_{2.5}$, and CO is associated with increased methylation of the Foxp3 gene promoter, which is significantly associated with asthma in adults.[79] Similarly, a 2017 meta-analysis demonstrated that higher concentrations of NO_2, $PM_{2.5}$ and sulfur dioxide (SO_2) were significantly associated with asthma exacerbation in children.[80,81] Thus, such findings are especially important for elementary and middle schools.

Schools have a unique indoor air pollutant environment, as there are relatively few airborne irritants that originate from within the school, given that fuel-burning kitchens and tobacco smoking is inhibited on school premises. However, the surrounding environment may be a prime source of airborne irritants. For example, 3.2 million US children attend school within 100 miles of a major highway.[82,83] Proximity to a major roadway is associated with greater asthma morbidity, likely due to road dust and primary traffic pollutants such as elemental carbon, fresh PM mass, ultrafine particles, and nitric oxide.[82,83] Additionally, cars and buses often idle outside schools for pick-up and drop-off twice a day, creating peak hours of exposure.[76,81] These factors are especially relevant to inner-city schools due to their proximity to highways and consistent heavy traffic.[80,81,83–85]

Nitrogen dioxide and ozone are the main components of urban smog. Gaffin and colleagues[7] studied the effect of indoor NO_2 exposure in inner-city schools and found that indoor classroom NO_2 was highly associated with increased airflow obstruction in inner-city children with asthma.

Increasing NO_2 exposure also worsened asthma symptoms for obese inner-city children with asthma.[86] Ozone may also cause susceptibility to inhaled allergens or toxins via ROS-disrupted epithelial integrity, thus promoting proinflammatory mediators.[7]

In a similar cohort, Gaffin and colleagues, 2017 explored school environmental exposures and identified relative source contributions of indoor and outdoor $PM_{2.5}$ for inner-city school classrooms. The study found outdoor PM sources come mainly from industrial or traffic-related combustion, while indoor PM sources arise from smoking and indoor cooking.[77] The main finding indicates that $PM_{2.5}$ has important classroom sources, which vary by school and site-specific outdoor PM levels.[77] These classroom $PM_{2.5}$ sources were upheld by Carrion-Matta and colleagues[81] in a subsequent SICAS study.

A recent SICAS investigation expands on Gaffin and colleagues 2017 by further examining factors that influence classroom exposures not only to $PM_{2.5}$, but to BC and NO_2 as well. Measurements of these pollutants over a 10-year period demonstrate that "regional" outdoor air pollution was the most important predictor of indoor $PM_{2.5}$, BC and NO_2.[87] School-based predictors included the presence of a furnace, a basement, the building type, the year in which it was built and ventilation method.[87] While classroom-based predictors included the classroom floor level, proximity to cafeteria, number of windows and number windows facing the bus area.[87] Identification of these influencing factors may inform target interventions aiming to improve children's school health. The effects of ventilation methods (natural, mixed, and mechanical) on school air pollutants were also investigated.[87] Schools which used natural ventilation practices (eg, winds and/or natural forces) were significantly and positively associated with classroom $PM_{2.5}$, again demonstrating that the most critical factor influencing classroom exposures is the infiltration of outdoor air pollutants.[87] The role of ventilation in augmenting classroom exposures was demonstrated in various schools across the United States and foreign countries.[87] Overall, mechanical or mixed ventilation systems equipped with HEPA filters or high-performance Minimum Efficiency Removal Value (MERV) filters are effective in removing common indoor allergens and reducing asthma symptoms.[88,89] Ventilation and proper air filtration can also reduce the risk of airborne disease transmission.[88,89] HEPA filters alone are at least 99.97% efficient at capturing COVID-19 associated particles, while studies show filtering room-air 5 times per hour can reduce risk of COVID-19 transmission by 50%.[89]

Therefore, future targeted interventions should consider the use of mechanical ventilation (e.g., fans) with attention to optimal air exchange rates and use of appropriate filters to effectively reduce the contribution of outdoor air pollution in schools, improve asthma symptoms and reduce the risk of viral transmission.[87–89]

There have been few school-based intervention studies on indoor air quality and health outcomes. In a randomized control trial of 19 primary schools in Australia, an intervention replacing unflued gas heaters with electric heaters significantly reduced the levels of NO_2 and asthma in the experimental group.[90] Also encouraging were the results of an intervention in which HEPA filters were installed in elementary school classrooms in the northeast United States. In intervention classrooms, $PM_{2.5}$ and BC were significantly reduced, and children demonstrated improvements in peak flow, but no significant changes in FEV_1 or asthma symptoms.[91]

School Environmental Intervention Studies and Challenges

Overall, more school-based studies examining environmental interventions and health outcomes are needed, especially in the United States. Few published European studies are large enough or adequately powered to comprehensively assess asthma morbidity outcomes.[12] The SICAS-2 intervention study has been among the first to conduct inner-city school interventions with the installment of classroom HEPA filters and school-wide IPM. The study revealed that HEPA filters significantly reduced airborne mouse and dog allergen, and that IPM reduced asthma symptoms early in the school, but overall, the benefit of interventions was not sustained.[21] Consideration of particle exposures, allergen levels, and asthma symptoms at baseline may be worthwhile.

It has been widely accepted that the school environment contains a large reservoir of exposures to environmental allergens–biologic and physical. It is evident that one intervention model may not be generalizable to all schools. Each school environment is uniquely its own, with variations in types of environmental exposures, geographic climate, socioeconomic conditions, and distance from highways and roadways, among other factors.[12,83,92] Although challenging, school-based environmental interventions have the potential to be highly beneficial to the health of the community at large, which includes children of school-age. Given this potential for significant national impact, additional research investigations and school mitigation strategies/programs could be ultimately cost-effective in addressing national health care utilization and individual families, by reducing disability, medical bills, hospital visits, unexpected days off work, and financial losses.

SUMMARY

A child's environment is critical in both the development and clinical course of asthma exacerbation. This review focuses on the most recent evidence supporting the role of the environment in asthma development, from biological and physical perspectives. With regard to future direction, it is important to investigate the critical exposure windows for asthma and allergen sensitization in pregnancy, early childhood, childhood, and adulthood through continued research and randomized controlled trials.[69] Health services research can be used to form the evidence-base needed by policy makers to enact change in schools and local communities. In the meantime, schools can follow currently established protocols to decrease asthma exposure risk outlined by the Indoor Air Quality (IAQ) Tools for Schools Action Kit to protect the health of school-aged children.[93]

CLINICS CARE POINTS

- Recommend intervention strategies for the reduction of common indoor allergen exposures. Strategies may largely be used in both the home and/or school settings. The effects of these interventions on asthma symptom improvement are variable, but are effective in reducing allergen/irritant exposure overall: *Cockroach:* IPM using insecticidal bait. *Mouse:* IPM including the use of sticky traps, blocking entry ways, removing possible sources of food/water, terminating pest count with low-toxicity pesticides. *Cat and Dog:* modify cats' diet using anti-Fel d 1 immunoglobulin Y, HEPA filters, HEPA integrated vacuums, and frequent washing of pets. *Dust Mite:* removal and/or washing of fabrics and upholstery, HEPA filters. *Fungus and Mold:* reduce moisture, increase ventilation, HEPA filters. *Microbiome:* improve composition through IPM. *Air pollution:* replacement of gas heaters with electric heaters, HEPA filters.

- Promote the use of the ADA policy and Section 504 of the Rehabilitation Act which requires schools to accommodate children with disabilities, including allergies. The allergist/immunologist can help facilitate a 504 plan and communicate with school administrators and nurses to develop an action plan for the school.

- Promote established protocols outlined by the Indoor Air Quality (IAQ) Tools for Schools Action Kit to build successful school-based asthma programs and asthma-friendly schools.

ACKNOWLEDGMENTS

Grant IDs:1. 5K24AI106822 2. 5U01AI126614 3. 5R01HL137192 4. 5UO1AI1103975. Co-Author Tina Banzon also has a NIH T32 grant which should be placed on the cover: NIH T32 AI7512-35.

DISCLOSURE

All authors do not have any financial and personal relationships with other people or organizations that could influence (bias) their work. The authors have no disclosures of any affiliation with any organization with a financial interest, direct or indirect, in the subject matter or materials discussed in the article (such as consultancies, employment, paid expert testimony, honoraria, speaker's bureaus, retainers, stock options or ownership, patents or patent applications or travel grants) that may affect the conduct or reporting of the work submitted.

REFERENCES

1. Allergy facts: allergies are the 6th leading cause of chronic illness in the U.S. In: ACAAI patient. 2022. Available at: https://acaai.org/allergies/allergies-101/facts-stats/. Accessed April 12, 2022.
2. Asthma. In: CDC National Center for Health Statistics. 2022. Available at: https://www.cdc.gov/nchs/fastats/asthma.htm. Accessed April 25, 2022.
3. Rubner FJ, Jackson DJ, Evans MD, et al. Early life rhinovirus wheezing, allergic sensitization, and asthma risk at adolescence. J Allergy Clin Immunol 2017; 139(2):501–7.
4. Klepeis NE, Nelson WC, Ott WR, et al. The National Human Activity Pattern Survey (NHAPS): a resource for assessing exposure to environmental pollutants. J Expo Sci Environ Epidemiol 2001;11(3):231–52.
5. Rosenstreich DL, Eggleston P, Kattan M, et al. The role of cockroach allergy and exposure to cockroach allergen in causing morbidity among inner-city children with asthma. N Engl J Med 1997;336(19):1356–63.
6. Crain EF, Walter M, O'Connor GT, et al. Home and allergic characteristics of children with asthma in seven U.S. urban communities and design of an environmental intervention: the inner-city asthma study. Environ Health Perspect 2002; 110(9):939–45.
7. Gaffin JM, Hauptman M, Petty CR, et al. Nitrogen dioxide exposure in school classrooms of inner-city children with asthma. J Allergy Clin Immunol 2018; 141(6):2249–55.e2.
8. Sheehan WJ, Permaul P, Petty CR, et al. Association Between Allergen Exposure in Inner-City Schools and Asthma Morbidity Among Students. JAMA Pediatr 2017;171(1):31–8.
9. Chen C-H, Chao HJ, Chan C-C, et al. Current asthma in schoolchildren is related to fungal spores in classrooms. Chest 2014;146(1):123–34.
10. Holst GJ, Høst A, Doekes G, et al. Allergy and respiratory health effects of dampness and dampness-related agents in schools and homes: a cross-sectional study in Danish pupils. Indoor Air 2016;26(6):880–91.
11. Almqvist C, Wickman M, Perfetti L, et al. Worsening of asthma in children allergic to cats, after indirect exposure to cat at school. Am J Respir Crit Care Med 2001; 163(3 Pt 1):694–8.
12. Esty B, Permaul P, DeLoreto K, et al. Asthma and allergies in the school environment. Clin Rev Allergy Immunol 2019;57(3):415–26.
13. Matsui EC, Wood RA, Rand C, et al. Cockroach allergen exposure and sensitization in suburban middle-class children with asthma. J Allergy Clin Immunol 2003; 112(1):87–92.
14. Pomés A, Mueller GA, Randall TA, et al. New insights into cockroach allergens. Curr Allergy Asthma Rep 2017;17(4):25.
15. Sheehan WJ, Rangsithienchai PA, Muilenberg ML, et al. Mouse allergens in urban elementary schools and homes of children with asthma. Ann Allergy Asthma Immunol 2009;102(2):125–30.

16. Satyaraj E, Wedner HJ, Bousquet J. Keep the cat, change the care pathway: a transformational approach to managing Fel d 1, the major cat allergen. Allergy 2019;74(Suppl 107):5–17.

17. Rabito FA, Carlson JC, He H, et al. A single intervention for cockroach control reduces cockroach exposure and asthma morbidity in children. J Allergy Clin Immunol 2017;140(2):565–70.

18. Portnoy J, Miller JD, Williams PB, et al. Environmental assessment and exposure control of dust mites: a practice parameter. Ann Allergy Asthma Immunol 2013; 111(6):465–507.

19. Morgan WJ, Gruchalla RS, Kattan M, et al. Results of a home-based environmental intervention among urban children with asthma. N Engl J Med 2004; 351:1068–80.

20. DiMango E, Serebrisky D, Narula S, et al. Individualized household allergen intervention lowers allergen level but not asthma medication use: a randomized controlled trial. J Allergy Clin Immunol Pract 2016;4(4):671–9.e4.

21. Phipatanakul W, Koutrakis P, Coull BA, et al. Effect of school integrated pest management or classroom air filter purifiers on asthma symptoms in students with active asthma: a randomized clinical trial. JAMA 2021;326(9):839.

22. Phipatanakul W, Eggleston PA, Wright EC, et al. Mouse allergen. I. The prevalence of mouse allergen in inner-city homes. The National Cooperative Inner-City Asthma Study. J Allergy Clin Immunol 2000;106(6):1070–4.

23. Matsui EC, Simons E, Rand C, et al. Airborne mouse allergen in the homes of inner-city children with asthma. J Allergy Clin Immunol 2005;115(2):358–63.

24. Phipatanakul W, Eggleston PA, Wright EC, et al. Mouse allergen. II. The relationship of mouse allergen exposure to mouse sensitization and asthma morbidity in inner-city children with asthma. J Allergy Clin Immunol 2000;106(6):1075–80.

25. Matsui EC, Wood RA, Rand C, et al. Mouse allergen exposure and mouse skin test sensitivity in suburban, middle-class children with asthma. J Allergy Clin Immunol 2004;113(5):910–5.

26. Cohn RD, Arbes SJ, Yin M, et al. National prevalence and exposure risk for mouse allergen in US households. J Allergy Clin Immunol 2004;113(6):1167–71.

27. Matsui EC, Perzanowski M, Peng RD, et al. Effect of an integrated pest management intervention on asthma symptoms among mouse-sensitized children and adolescents with asthma: a randomized clinical trial. JAMA 2017;317(10): 1027–36.

28. Szefler S, Weiss S, Tonascia J, et al. Long-term effects of budesonide or nedocromil in children with asthma. N Engl J Med 2000;343(15):1054–63.

29. Akar-Ghibril N, Sheehan WJ, Perzanowski M, et al. Predictors of successful mouse allergen reduction in inner-city homes of children with asthma. J Allergy Clin Immunol Pract 2021;9(11):4159–61.e2.

30. Phipatanakul W, Bailey A, Hoffman EB, et al. The school inner-city asthma study (SICAS): design, methods, and lessons learned. J Asthma 2011;48(10):1007–14.

31. Busse WW, Jackson DJ. School classrooms as targets to reduce allergens and improve asthma. JAMA 2021;326(9):816–7.

32. Ingram JM, Sporik R, Rose G, et al. Quantitative assessment of exposure to dog (Can f 1) and cat (Fel d 1) allergens: relation to sensitization and asthma among children living in Los Alamos, New Mexico. J Allergy Clin Immunol 1995;96(4): 449–56.

33. Custovic A, Fletcher A, Pickering CA, et al. Domestic allergens in public places III: house dust mite, cat, dog and cockroach allergens in British hospitals. Clin Exp Allergy 1998;28(1):53–9.

34. Springer J. The 2021-2022 APPA National pet owners survey statistics: pet ownership & annual expenses. In: American pet products association. 2022. Available from: https://www.americanpetproducts.org/press_industrytrends.asp. Accessed April, 19 2022.

35. De Lucca SD, O'meara TJ, Tovey ER. Exposure to mite and cat allergens on a range of clothing items at home and the transfer of cat allergen in the workplace. J Allergy Clin Immunol 2000;106(5):874–9.

36. Karlsson A-S, Renström A. Human hair is a potential source of cat allergen contamination of ambient air. Allergy 2005;60(7):961–4.

37. Perzanowski MS, Ronmark E, James HR, et al. Relevance of specific IgE antibody titer to the prevalence, severity, and persistence of asthma among 19-year-olds in northern Sweden. J Allergy Clin Immunol 2016;138(6):1582–90.

38. Salo PM, Sever ML, Zeldin DC. Indoor allergens in school and daycare environments. J Allergy Clin Immunol 2009;124(2):185–94.

39. Perzanowski MS, Rönmark E, Nold B, et al. Relevance of allergens from cats and dogs to asthma in the northernmost province of Sweden: schools as a major site of exposure. J Allergy Clin Immunol 1999;103(6):1018–24.

40. Krop EJM, Jacobs JH, Sander I, et al. "Allergens and β-Glucans in Dutch Homes and Schools: Characterizing Airborne Levels." PLOS ONE 9, no. 2: e88871. https://doi.org/10.1371/journal.pone.0088871.

41. Maciag MC, Phipatanakul W. Update on indoor allergens and their impact on pediatric asthma. Ann Allergy Asthma Immunol 2022;(0). https://doi.org/10.1016/j.anai.2022.02.009.

42. Permaul P, Hoffman E, Fu C, et al. Allergens in urban schools and homes of children with asthma. Pediatr Allergy Immunol 2012;23(6):543–9.

43. Rud AG, Beck AM. Companion animals in Indiana elementary schools. Anthrozoos 2003;16(3):241–51.

44. Ganzert RR, McCullough A. Pets in the classroom study: phase I findings report. In: American Humane association. 2015. Available at: https://www.americanhumane.org/publication/pets-in-the-classroom-study-phase-i-findings-report/. Accessed April 29, 2022.

45. Arlian LG, Bernstein D, Bernstein IL, et al. Prevalence of dust mites in the homes of people with asthma living in eight different geographic areas of the United States. J Allergy Clin Immunol 1992;90(3 Pt 1):292–300.

46. Kanchongkittiphon W, Mendell MJ, Gaffin JM, et al. Indoor environmental exposures and exacerbation of asthma: an update to the 2000 review by the Institute of Medicine. Environ Health Perspect 2015;123(1):6–20.

47. Platts-Mills TAE, Vervloet D, Thomas WR, et al. Indoor allergens and asthma:Report of the Third International Workshop. J Allergy Clin Immunol 1997;100(6):S2–24.

48. Platts-Mills TAE, de Weck AL, Aalberse RC, et al. Dust mite allergens and asthma—A worldwide problem. J Allergy Clin Immunol 1989;83(2, Part 1):416–27.

49. Zock JP, Brunekreef B. House dust mite allergen levels in dust from schools with smooth and carpeted classroom floors. Clin Exp Allergy 1995;25(6):549–53.

50. Fernández-Caldas E, Codina R, Ledford DK, et al. House dust mite, cat, and cockroach allergen concentrations in daycare centers in Tampa, Florida. Ann Allergy Asthma Immunol 2001;87(3):196–200.

51. Choi S-Y, Lee I-Y, Sohn J-H, et al. Optimal conditions for the removal of house dust mite, dog dander, and pollen allergens using mechanical laundry. Ann Allergy Asthma Immunol 2008;100(6):583–8.

52. McDonald LG, Tovey E. The role of water temperature and laundry procedures in reducing house dust mite populations and allergen content of bedding. J Allergy Clin Immunol 1992;90(4 Pt 1):599–608.

53. Wilson JM, Platts-Mills TAE. Home Environmental Interventions for House Dust Mite. J Allergy Clin Immunol Pract 2018;6(1):1–7.

54. Murray CS, Foden P, Sumner H, et al. Preventing severe asthma exacerbations in children. A randomized trial of mite-impermeable bedcovers. Am J Respir Crit Care Med 2017;196(2):150–8.

55. Fisk WJ, Lei-Gomez Q, Mendell MJ. Meta-analyses of the associations of respiratory health effects with dampness and mold in homes. Indoor Air 2007;17(4): 284–96.

56. Gent JF, Kezik JM, Hill ME, et al. Household mold and dust allergens: exposure, sensitization and childhood asthma morbidity. Environ Res 2012;118:86–93.

57. Karvonen AM, Hyvärinen A, Korppi M, et al. Moisture damage and asthma: a birth cohort study. Pediatrics 2015;135(3):e598–606.

58. Mendell MJ, Mirer AG, Cheung K, et al. Respiratory and allergic health effects of dampness, mold, and dampness-related agents: a review of the epidemiologic evidence. Environ Health Perspect 2011;119(6):748–56.

59. Quansah R, Jaakkola MS, Hugg TT, et al. Residential dampness and molds and the risk of developing asthma: a systematic review and meta-analysis. PLoS One 2012;7(11):e47526.

60. Baxi SN, Sheehan WJ, Sordillo JE, et al. Association between fungal spore exposure in inner-city schools and asthma morbidity. Ann Allergy Asthma Immunol 2019;122(6):610–5.e1.

61. Simoni M, Cai G-H, Norback D, et al. Total viable molds and fungal DNA in classrooms and association with respiratory health and pulmonary function of European schoolchildren. Pediatr Allergy Immunol 2011;22(8):843–52.

62. Cavaleiro Rufo J, Madureira J, Paciência I, et al. Indoor fungal diversity in primary schools may differently influence allergic sensitization and asthma in children. Pediatr Allergy Immunol 2017;28(4):332–9.

63. Kercsmar CM, Dearborn DG, Schluchter M, et al. Reduction in asthma morbidity in children as a result of home remediation aimed at moisture sources. Environ Health Perspect 2006;114(10):1574–80.

64. Sauni R, Uitti J, Jauhiainen M, et al. Remediating buildings damaged by dampness and mould for preventing or reducing respiratory tract symptoms, infections and asthma. Cochrane Database Syst Rev 2011;(9): CD007897.

65. Baxi SN, Muilenberg ML, Rogers CA, et al. Exposures to Molds in School Classrooms of Children with Asthma. Pediatr Allergy Immunol 2013;24(7):697–703.

66. Howard EJ, Vesper SJ, Guthrie BJ, et al. Asthma prevalence and mold levels in US northeastern schools. J Allergy Clin Immunol Pract 2021;9(3): 1312–8.

67. Vesper S, McKinstry C, Haugland R, et al. Development of an environmental relative moldiness index for US homes. J Occup Environ Med 2007;49(8): 829–33.

68. Vesper SJ, Wymer L, Coull BA, et al. HEPA filtration intervention in classrooms may improve some students' asthma. J Asthma 2022;1–8.

69. Louisias M, Ramadan A, Naja AS, et al. The effects of the environment on asthma disease activity. Immunol Allergy Clin N Am 2019;39(2):163–75.

70. Lai PS, Kolde R, Franzosa EA, et al. The classroom microbiome and asthma morbidity in children attending three inner-city schools. J Allergy Clin Immunol 2018;141(6):2311-3.

71. Gauderman WJ, Urman R, Avol E, et al. Association of improved air quality with lung development in children. N Engl J Med 2015;372(10):905-13.

72. Strickland MJ, Darrow LA, Klein M, et al. Short-term associations between ambient air pollutants and pediatric asthma emergency department visits. Am J Respir Crit Care Med 2010;182(3):307-16.

73. Silverman RA, Ito K. Age-related association of fine particles and ozone with severe acute asthma in New York City. J Allergy Clin Immunol 2010;125(2):367-73.e5.

74. Effects of air pollution on children's health and development. In: World Health Organization. 2005. Available at: https://www.euro.who.int/__data/assets/pdf_file/0010/74728/E86575.pdf. Accessed April 15, 2022.

75. Mannucci PM, Harari S, Martinelli I, et al. Effects on health of air pollution: a narrative review. Intern Emerg Med 2015;10(6):657-62.

76. Hochstetler HA, Yermakov M, Reponen T, et al. Aerosol particles generated by diesel-powered school buses at urban schools as a source of children's exposure. Atmos Environ (1994) 2011;45(7):1444-53.

77. Gaffin JM, Petty CR, Hauptman M, et al. Modeling indoor particulate exposures in inner-city school classrooms. J Expo Sci Environ Epidemiol 2017;27(5):451-7.

78. Keet CA, Keller JP, Peng RD. Long-term coarse particulate matter exposure is associated with asthma among children in medicaid. Am J Respir Crit Care Med 2018;197(6):737-46.

79. Prunicki M, Stell L, Dinakarpandian D, et al. Exposure to NO2, CO, and PM2.5 is linked to regional DNA methylation differences in asthma. Clin Epigenetics 2018;10:2.

80. Naja AS, Permaul P, Phipatanakul W. Taming asthma in school-aged children: a comprehensive review. J Allergy Clin Immunol Pract 2018;6(3):726-35.

81. Carrion-Matta A, Kang C-M, Gaffin JM, et al. Classroom indoor PM2.5 sources and exposures in inner-city schools. Environ Int 2019;131:104968.

82. Kingsley SL, Eliot MN, Carlson L, et al. Proximity of US schools to major roadways: a nationwide assessment. J Expo Sci Environ Epidemiol 2014;24(3):253-9.

83. Hauptman M, Gaffin JM, Petty CR, et al. Proximity to major roadways and asthma symptoms in the School Inner-City Asthma Study. J Allergy Clin Immunol 2020;145(1):119-26.e4.

84. Pollock J, Shi L, Gimbel RW. Outdoor environment and pediatric asthma: an update on the evidence from North America. Can Respir J 2017;2017:8921917.

85. Yoda Y, Takagi H, Wakamatsu J, et al. Acute effects of air pollutants on pulmonary function among students: a panel study in an isolated island. Environ Health Prev Med 2017;22(1):33.

86. Permaul P, Gaffin JM, Petty CR, et al. Obesity may enhance the adverse effects of NO2 exposure in urban schools on asthma symptoms in children. J Allergy Clin Immunol 2020;146(4):813-20.e2.

87. Matthaios VN, Kang C-M, Wolfson JM, et al. Factors influencing classroom exposures to fine particles, black carbon, and nitrogen dioxide in inner-city schools and their implications for indoor air quality. Environ Health Perspect 2022;130(4):47005.

88. Brown KW, Minegishi T, Allen JG, et al. Reducing patients' exposures to asthma and allergy triggers in their homes: an evaluation of effectiveness of grades of forced air ventilation filters. J Asthma 2014;51(6):585–94.
89. Let's Clear The Air On COVID. In: The white house. 2022. Available at: https://www.whitehouse.gov/ostp/news-updates/2022/03/23/lets-clear-the-air-on-covid. Accessed May 17, 2022.
90. Pilotto LS, Nitschke M, Smith BJ, et al. Randomized controlled trial of unflued gas heater replacement on respiratory health of asthmatic schoolchildren. Int J Epidemiol 2004;33(1):208–14.
91. Jhun I, Gaffin JM, Coull BA, et al. School environmental intervention to reduce particulate pollutant exposures for children with asthma. J Allergy Clin Immunol Pract 2017;5(1):154–9.e3.
92. Permaul P, Phipatanakul W. School environmental intervention programs. J Allergy Clin Immunol Pract 2018;6(1):22–9.
93. Indoor Air Quality Tools for Schools in Action Kit. In: United States Environmental Protection Agency. 2021. Available at: https://www.epa.gov/iaq-schools/indoor-air-quality-tools-schools-action-kit. Accessed on April 19, 2022.

Eosinophilic Esophagitis
The Role of Environmental Exposures

Mehr Zahra Shah, MD[a], Brooke I. Polk, MD[b],*

KEYWORDS

- Eosinophilic esophagitis • Microbiome • Exposome • Environmental exposure

KEY POINTS

- Eosinophilic esophagitis is a chronic, non-immunoglobulin E (IgE) immune-mediated disease, which is clinicopathologically characterized by eosinophilic infiltration and presents with symptoms of esophageal dysfunction.
- Pathogenesis of the disease is thought to be multifactorial, likely a combination of prenatal and early life exposures, genetics, exposome, and aeroallergens.
- The developing immune system, and subsequently the host microbiome, is shaped by early life exposures. Lack of early life exposures to pathogens results in immune tolerance defects and alters the host microbiome which drives microbiota toward a T-helper 2 phenotype.
- Studies are showing seasonal variation in eosinophilic esophagitis (EoE) diagnosis and flares point toward environmental allergen involvement. EoE can develop after a large identifiable aeroallergen exposure.
- EoE is more common in rural areas with low population density, which seems counterintuitive to other atopic diseases.

BACKGROUND

Eosinophilic esophagitis (EoE) is a chronic inflammatory condition characterized by esophageal dysfunction with potential for fibrotic remodeling. Within the past two decades, EoE has emerged as a major cause for esophageal morbidity, with rapidly rising incidence and prevalence.[1] Atopic comorbidities are common in EoE, and similar cytokines are activated across type 2 inflammatory processes, suggesting a shared pathogenesis involving impaired epithelial integrity.[2] Although food allergens play a clear role in the development of EoE, the full disease process remains poorly understood. Not all EoE patients respond to dietary therapy, with up to 10% not

a Washington University in Saint Louis School of Medicine, 660 South Euclid Avenue, St Louis, MO 63110, USA; b Division of Allergy and Pulmonary Medicine, Washington University in Saint Louis School of Medicine, 1 Children's Place, Mail Stop 8116-43-14, Campus box 8116, St Louis, MO 63110, USA
* Corresponding author.
E-mail address: bpolk@wustl.edu

Immunol Allergy Clin N Am 42 (2022) 761–770
https://doi.org/10.1016/j.iac.2022.05.006
0889-8561/22/© 2022 Elsevier Inc. All rights reserved.

achieving remission with an elemental diet in a large meta-analysis.[3] This suggests that, at least for a subset of patients with EoE, another trigger exists. Recent epidemiologic and clinical studies suggest the involvement of external environmental influences in at least some individuals with EoE.[4]

The developing immune system is critically susceptible to external factors, and the emerging field of exposomics seeks to understand how lifetime environmental exposures affect health.[5]

Exposure to biologic and chemical insults such as allergen proteases, detergents, ozone, and particulate matter damages the epithelial barrier, potentially leading to chronic inflammation.[6]

This article summarizes recent data demonstrating the integral role of environmental factors in the development and ongoing inflammatory pathway of EoE. We also discuss current gaps in knowledge regarding EoE and the environment.

EARLY LIFE EXPOSURES AND THE HYGIENE HYPOTHESIS

Predisposition to EoE is thought to consist of a complex interplay of environmental factors such as early life exposures, diet, geography, modifiable risk factors, and epigenetics (**Fig. 1**).[7] The recent increase in incidence has led to multiple case control studies looking into these exposures and their association with EoE.

One single-center case control study enrolling over 100 participants investigated these factors further and found that prenatal exposures, such as maternal fever, preterm labor, and Cesarean delivery, and early life exposures such as antibiotic and acid suppression in infancy, were all associated with an increased risk of EoE.[8] These early life events may lead to decreased exposure to microbes and consequently an under-challenged immune system during a critical time in immune system development, resulting in dysbiosis. During pregnancy, maternal fever generates proinflammatory cytokines that disrupt the development of the fetal immune system and consequently predispose to EoE. Other exposures such as Neonatal Intensive Care Unit (NICU) admission and antibiotic exposure disrupt immune system development by altering gut colonization, which is essential for not only establishing a mucosal barrier but also promoting immune system maturation. These factors are each understood to negatively impact the immune system formation during a critical time.[8]

These associations are further highlighted by analyzing patients with very early onset EoE (V-EoE), those who develop EoE within the first 12 months of life. A single-center retrospective study (n = 57) examined factors associated with V-EoE to better understand the etiology of the disease and found that Cesarean delivery

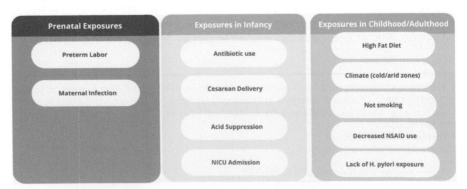

Fig. 1. Environmental exposures associated with EoE.

was more common in V-EoE.[9] Cesarean delivery is thought to alter the development of the patient's microbiome because patients are not exposed to vaginal microflora, which in turn affects the immune system and predisposes to EoE development.

Acid suppression in infancy has also been positively associated with EoE. A retrospective cohort study by Kuhn and colleagues[10] found a statistically significant positive association between proton-pump inhibitor (PPI) usage (5.7% vs 1.6%, $P < .0001$) and H2-antagonist usage (8.8% vs 4.5%, $P < .0001$) and EoE. This is an interesting finding given that PPIs are often used for the treatment of EoE once the diagnosis is established. This association may be explained by the barrier disruption and alteration in digestion cause by PPIs. PPIs inhibit the digestion of food proteins, which leads to the absorption of larger intact proteins, generating an immune response and potential development of IgE antibodies against food proteins.[11] A recall survey of 127 children with EoE and 121 controls showed further association, with reported acid suppression use in infancy associated with EoE and adjusted odds ratio (aOR) 7.41.[8] Although these studies only point to association rather than causation, this is an area that warrants further exploration.

Diet has also been explored as a potential trigger. Although research is still nascent, one study by Silva and colleagues[12] found that high-fat diet (HFD)-induced obesity increased T-helper 2 (TH2) immune responses in EoE murine models. The results were supported by Gu and colleagues,[13] who suggested that HFD leads to mucosal barrier disruption, possibly via peroxisome proliferator-activated receptor gamma (PPAR-χ)-induced inflammation. In addition to being the master transcriptional regulator of adipogenesis, PPAR-χ promotes interleukin-33 receptor expression on TH2 cells and type 2 innate lymphoid cells, driving increased responsiveness to the alarmin IL-33 and thus activation of the type 2 allergic response.[14] PPAR-χ is certainly an interesting potential therapeutic target in TH2 diseases.

Geographic region and weather have also been investigated for their role in EoE. A cross-sectional epidemiologic study showed variation in esophageal eosinophilia based on different Koppen–Geiger (K–G) climate zones. K–G climate zone classification system allocates by geographic location and includes factors such as climate type, precipitation, and monthly temperatures. The study found that cold and arid K–G climate zones were found to have the highest prevalence of EoE.[15] Although the reason is unclear, one hypothesis is that aeroallergens within different geographic climate zones likely play a role in the development in EoE. Namely, the flora within these regions generates more potent airborne antigens than those in tropical zones. Studies exploring the relationship between EoE and aeroallergens will be discussed further in this article.

One notable aspect of EoE is the observation that EoE is more common in rural areas as compared with urban areas, and population density is strongly and inversely associated with EoE.[16] Within a cross-sectional case control study of a US pathology database (n = 292,621), individuals living in the lowest quintile of population density were at significantly higher odds of having an endoscopy with greater than 15 eosinophils/high-powered field (hpf), compared with those in the highest quintile (aOR 1.27 [1.18–1.36]).[16] With higher esophageal eosinophil counts, the inverse relationship strengthened. This finding is counterintuitive given that most atopic diseases are more prevalent in urban settings due to multifactorial explanations including urban pollutants, sanitation, and decreased exposure to microbes.[17] This observation lends itself to more investigation on exposures present within rural areas which may be relevant in the mechanism of predisposition to EoE, such as exposure to livestock, pesticides, outdoor allergen concentration, or differences in particulate matter seasonal variations in EoE may be important but remain under investigation.[18]

Other environmental factors impacting EoE may be modifiable. For example, one case control study of 115 cases and 225 controls demonstrated that current non-steroidal anti inflammatory drug (NSAID) use (17% vs 40%, $P < .001$) and ever having smoked cigarettes (23% vs 47%, $P < .001$) were inversely associated with EoE. Although alcohol use was more prevalent in EoE, it was not an independent risk factor for EoE development. There was a trend toward histologic improvement in EoE patients concomitantly taking NSAIDs (87% vs 63%, $P = .08$).[19] Factors with a potential protective association against EoE are indoor pets and *Helicobacter pylori* infection, both of which may be explained by the hygiene hypothesis.[18]

Current research shows that heritability is more pronounced with the influence of strong environmental cues as well as weaker genetic cues.[20] However, the role environmental exposures have on modifying genes or impacting EoE pathogenesis/diagnosis is unclear. The interplay of EoE-predisposing polymorphisms in Calpain 14 (CAPN14) and LOC283710/KLF13 genes and early life environment factors might contribute to EoE susceptibility. A recent case analysis identified interactions between the rs6736278 CAPN14 polymorphism and breastfeeding ($P = .02$) and between the rs17815905 KLF13 polymorphism and NICU admission ($P = .02$). Subsequent case-control analysis showed that breastfeeding reduced the risk of EoE development in those with the CAPN14 single nucleotide polymorphism (SNP) (aOR 0.08 [0.01–0.59]).[21] An earlier mentioned study analyzing factors associated with V-EoE showed that those with V-EoE share genetic factors including enrichment in CAPN14 gene loci.[9] Effect modification at these genetic variants highlights the gene-environment interplay that also plays a role in the development of the disease. Further studies on epigenetics and EoE may shed more light on having certain genetic variants and the response when these exposed to these environmental factors.

HOST MICROBIOME

An investigation into predisposition to EoE would be remiss without discussion of the microbiome. The role of the microbiome in the development of EoE is rooted in the hygiene hypothesis, which essentially states that lack of childhood infections results in a defect in immune tolerance and subsequent development of allergic disease. This leads to microbial dysbiosis and may explain the recent increase of EoE.[22]

This alteration in the microbiome generates a variety of inflammatory markers and increases serum IgE, serum basophils, and TH2 response in murine models.[23,24] One factor that has been shown to play a role in EoE is *H pylori* infection. Several studies have shown an inverse relationship between *H pylori* and EoE, though none prove causation.[25,26] A large meta-analysis of 11 observational studies (n = 377,795) found that *H pylori* exposure yielded a 37% reduction in EoE risk (OR 0.63 [0.51–0.78].[26] The proposed etiology for this association is *H pylori* virulence factors such as cytotoxic-associated gene A (CagA), vacuolating cytotoxin A (VacA), and gamma-glutamyl transpeptidase, which may attenuate regulatory T cells and/or cause TH1 polarization.[26] A recent review article calls the protective effect of *H pylori* into question, noting methodologic limitations of prior studies, including the retrospective nature of most studies.[27] A 2018 prospective case-control study (n = 808) of children and adults with EoE found no difference in *H pylori* prevalence in cases versus controls (37% vs 40%, $P = .3$ OR 0.97 [0.73–1.30]).[28]

Previous studies held that the esophagus contained few pathogens. However, with the increase of throughput data, gene sequencing revealed the richness of the esophageal microbiome with over 300 bacterial species.[29] One study conducted in pediatric patients found that a healthy control cohort had more diversity than those with EoE, but this did not reach statistical significance likely due to low power (*n* = 41).[30] Another smaller cohort study conducted in adults (n = 21) did not show any significant differences in the esophageal microbiome between those with EoE and without EoE.[31] The saliva has also been shown to have a diverse composition and differences in patients with EoE. Those with EoE were found to have a higher burden of *Haernophilus* species, which also had a positive association with disease activity.[23] In a murine model of EoE, neonatal antibiotic administration reduced the abundance of *Lactobacillales* and exaggerated the TH2 immune response; fecal microbiome transplant restored the esophageal microbiota in this model.[32]

Given the differences seen in the esophageal microbiome of EoE, studies have also investigated the effects of food triggers on the esophageal microbiome. Benitez and colleagues compared oral and esophageal microbiome differences and found an increased amount of *Proteobacteriae* in those with EoE versus increased *Streptococcus* in control groups. In addition, they evaluated how food elimination affected the microbiome, although elimination failed to produce significant changes, reintroduction of certain foods altered the microbiome, with increased *Granulicatella* and *Campylobacter* genera.[33]

Gene sequencing has provided a rich amount of data on the microbiome, and it is anticipated that future studies will provide additional information on whether alterations in the microbiome are due to EoE pathogenesis or esophageal inflammation in general. Furthermore, more research is needed to evaluate the multifactorial relationship between gene expression and the microbiome; metaproteomics may allow for targeted therapies, potentially focusing on gene therapy.[24]

AEROALLERGENS AND EOSINOPHILIC ESOPHAGITIS

With incidence and prevalence on the increase, EoE is now considered a late manifestation of the atopic march. In a longitudinal birth cohort study of 139 children with EoE, the presence of atopic dermatitis (Hazard ratio (HR) 3.2, 95% CI 2.2–4.6), IgE-mediated food allergy (HR 9.1, 95% CI 6.5–12.6), and asthma (HR 1.9, 95% CI 1.3–2.7) were independently associated with a diagnosis of EoE. In addition, the presence of EoE was associated with subsequent diagnosis of allergic rhinitis (HR 2.5, 95% CI 1.7–3.5).[34] Sensitization to aeroallergens is common in EoE, though it remains unclear whether aeroallergens are causal in EoE pathogenesis.[35]

A role for environmental allergens in EoE pathogenesis was first postulated in 2001 in animal models when Mishra and colleagues exposed anesthetized mice to repeated challenges of *Aspergillus fumigatus* aeroallergen; with respiratory exposure, mice had not only was airway inflammation but also a marked esophageal eosinophilia. Interleukin-5 was shown to be integral in esophageal eosinophil accumulation, as mice deficient in IL-5 had a markedly reduced esophageal reaction to *A fumigatus* spores. Esophageal eosinophilia developed only when sensitized mice were challenged intranasally and not via oral or intragastric allergen instillation.[36] Similar findings were demonstrated with allergen challenge with cockroach and dust mite allergens.[37] Subsequent murine studies showed that epicutaneous exposure to *A fumigatus* can also trigger EoE.[38]

Corresponding to these earlier animal studies demonstrating a role for aeroallergens in EoE, Wolf and colleagues[39] reported on a case series in 2013 in which *de novo* EoE developed in three patients following real-world large-volume aeroallergen exposure to grass pollen and mold spores. Unfortunately, follow-up was only available on one subject, in whom endoscopy confirmed resolution of EoE with aeroallergen removal. Intentional sublingual exposure to aeroallergens also seems to be a trigger in some individuals with EoE, with case reports demonstrating biopsy-confirmed induction of EoE by sublingual immunotherapy (SLIT) to tree, grass, and dust mite extracts.[40–43] The first case was demonstrated in 2003 by Miehlke and colleagues[41] in a 44 year old woman with allergic rhinoconjunctivitis undergoing SLIT to tree pollen, with complete resolution 4 weeks after SLIT cessation and no other interventions. In another case, EoE developed in a child completely dependent on enteral elemental gastrostomy feedings 1 month after starting pollen and dust mite SLIT, with clinical and endoscopic evidence of resolution following the discontinuation of SLIT therapy.[42]

Several studies have demonstrated seasonal variation in both the diagnosis and disease activity of EoE, suggesting a causal role in some patients, though results are not replicated consistently.[29,44–47] A single-center study of all patients with food impaction found significantly higher incidence in summer and fall months in patients with atopy and/or known EoE.[48] In a study of 234 children with EoE, Wang and colleagues[47] found that significantly fewer children were diagnosed with EoE in the winter months, and mean eosinophil burden was lower in the winter as well. In a large retrospective case series of patients (N = 160) with suspected aeroallergen-triggered EoE by history, 32 (20%) had biopsy-confirmed seasonal variations in eosinophil count. All 32 of these patients had allergic rhinitis.[45] However, reports of seasonal exacerbations in EoE patients in remission were uncommon in another cohort, with only 13 of 782 (4%) experiencing seasonal esophageal eosinophilia with no change in therapy.[46] A large meta-analysis of 16,846 patients with EoE found no statistical significance in seasonality of EoE diagnosis ($P = .132$) nor in exacerbations ($P = .699$).[49]

Interestingly, aeroallergen sensitization may play a role in response to EoE therapies. A link between EoE food triggers and pollen food allergy syndrome (PFAS) has been suggested. Twenty-five percent of adults with EoE patients reported PFAS in a recent cohort study.[50] Those with PFAS were less likely to respond to elimination diet and were more likely to have spring diagnoses of EoE. In a study of 123 individuals with EoE not responsive to PPI therapy, those with perennial allergen and mold sensitization were more likely to have nonresponse to combination therapy with diet and swallowed steroids.[51]

For some with EoE, limited case studies show that aeroallergen subcutaneous allergen immunotherapy (SCIT) may help achieve remission. Ramirez and colleagues[52] reported a 4-year-old boy with allergic rhinitis to dust mite and EoE recalcitrant to PPI, swallowed steroids, and elimination diet. Maintenance SCIT to dust mite resolved EoE, and the patient remained in remission at 4 years. A case report demonstrated success of multiallergen SCIT as monotherapy in inducing and maintaining complete clinical and histologic remission in a polysensitized teen boy with EoE, allergic rhinoconjunctivitis, and shellfish allergy who did not respond to standard therapies.[53]

SUMMARY/FUTURE DIRECTION

Given EoEs recent increase in incidence, further research is needed exploring its etiology to develop better management plans. As described here, environmental exposures seem to play an important role in the development of EoE. Research so far has shown that certain prenatal and early life exposures have a positive association with EoE, and these exposures can affect an individual differently depending on the individual's underlying genetic susceptibilities.[54] Furthermore, these early life exposures alter host microbiome development, thereby playing a role in altering immune system tolerance.[55] Several studies have shown these associations, but more research is needed in each of these areas to develop more targeted individualized therapies.

Although there have been many studies analyzing early life exposures, research is lacking on the role of various environmental factors such as aeroallergens and the association with EoE.

The current available evidence suggests that aeroallergens play a major role in some patients with EoE and at least a minor role in others. More research is important to understand the role of aeroallergens to reduce the disease burden through therapies targeting modifiable environmental factors.[55]

The future of EoE research depends on analyzing these environmental exposures and interlay of genetics to develop targeted therapies. In Europe, there is a registry study called EoE CONNECT, with the sole purpose of looking into clinical aspects of EoE and the different current therapies.[56] Such registries help provide more data for research analyzing exposures and triggers, which is essential to the development of future management plans for EoE.

CLINICS CARE POINTS

- Obtain a detailed history about patient's prenatal and early life exposures such as preterm labor, Cesarean delivery, NICU admission, and acid suppression in infancy. These early life exposures play a role in affecting the microbiome and further investigation into this may prevent atopic disorders.

- Various studies have shown a relationship between environment and eosinophilic esophagitis (EoE). It is important to include a patient's environment during history taking and when developing management plans for patients.

- Genetics also plays a role in EoE risk. More research is needed, but genetic panels may help serve as decision support tools for diagnosis and targeted therapies in the future.

- Currently, there is a lack of strong data on the impact of the environment on EoE. More research is still needed to better understand the number of patients with environment as their only trigger for EoE and also how the environment contributes to EoE symptoms.

DISCLOSURE

The authors have nothing to disclose.

REFERENCES

1. Dellon ES, Hirano I. Epidemiology and natural history of eosinophilic esophagitis. Gastroenterology 2018;154(2):319–32.e3.
2. Capucilli P, Hill DA. Allergic Comorbidity in Eosinophilic Esophagitis: Mechanistic Relevance and Clinical Implications. Clin Rev Allergy Immunol 2019;57(1): 111–27.
3. Warners MJ, Vlieg-Boerstra BJ, Bredenoord AJ. Elimination and elemental diet therapy in eosinophilic oesophagitis. Best Pract Res Clin Gastroenterol 2015; 29(5):793–803.
4. Furuta GT. Eosinophils in the esophagus: acid is not the only cause. J Pediatr Gastroenterol Nutr 1998;26(4):468–71.
5. Cecchi L, D'Amato G, Annesi-Maesano I. External exposome and allergic respiratory and skin diseases. J Allergy Clin Immunol 2018;141(3):846–57.
6. Celebi Sozener Z, Cevhertas L, Nadeau K, et al. Environmental factors in epithelial barrier dysfunction. J Allergy Clin Immunol 2020;145(6):1517–28.

7. Jensen ET, Dellon ES. Environmental factors and eosinophilic esophagitis. J Allergy Clin Immunol 2018;142(1):32–40.

8. Jensen ET, Kuhl JT, Martin LJ, et al. Prenatal, intrapartum, and postnatal factors are associated with pediatric eosinophilic esophagitis. J Allergy Clin Immunol 2017. https://doi.org/10.1016/j.jaci.2017.05.018.

9. Lyles JL, Martin LJ, Shoda T, et al. Very early onset eosinophilic esophagitis is common, responds to standard therapy, and demonstrates enrichment for CAPN14 genetic variants. J Allergy Clin Immunol 2021;147(1):244–254 e6.

10. Kuhn BR, Young AJ, Justice AE, et al. Infant acid suppression use is associated with the development of eosinophilic esophagitis. Dis Esophagus 2020;33(10): doaa073.

11. Trikha A, Baillargeon JG, Kuo YF, et al. Development of food allergies in patients with gastroesophageal reflux disease treated with gastric acid suppressive medications. Pediatr Allergy Immunol 2013;24(6):582–8.

12. Silva F, Oliveira EE, Ambrosio MGE, et al. High-fat diet-induced obesity worsens TH2 immune response and immunopathologic characteristics in murine model of eosinophilic oesophagitis. Clin Exp Allergy 2020;50(2):244–55.

13. Gu Y, Guo X, Sun S, et al. High-fat diet-induced obesity aggravates food allergy by intestinal barrier destruction and inflammation. Int Arch Allergy Immunol 2022; 183(1):80–92.

14. Stark JM, Coquet JM, Tibbitt CA. The Role of PPAR-gamma in Allergic Disease. Curr Allergy Asthma Rep 2021;21(11):45.

15. Hurrell JM, Genta RM, Dellon ES. Prevalence of esophageal eosinophilia varies by climate zone in the United States. Am J Gastroenterol 2012;107(5):698–706.

16. Jensen ET, Hoffman K, Shaheen NJ, et al. Esophageal eosinophilia is increased in rural areas with low population density: results from a national pathology database. Am J Gastroenterol 2014;109(5):668–75.

17. Stein MM, Hrusch CL, Gozdz J, et al. Innate Immunity and Asthma Risk in Amish and Hutterite Farm Children. N Engl J Med 2016;375(5):411–21.

18. Clayton F, Peterson K. Eosinophilic Esophagitis: Pathophysiology and Definition. Gastrointest Endosc Clin N Am 2018;28(1):1–14.

19. Koutlas NT, Eluri S, Rusin S, et al. Impact of smoking, alcohol consumption, and NSAID use on risk for and phenotypes of eosinophilic esophagitis. Dis Esophagus 2018;31(1):1–7.

20. Alexander ES, Martin LJ, Collins MH, et al. Twin and family studies reveal strong environmental and weaker genetic cues explaining heritability of eosinophilic esophagitis. J Allergy Clin Immunol 2014;134(5):1084–10892 e1.

21. Jensen ET, Kuhl JT, Martin LJ, et al. Early-life environmental exposures interact with genetic susceptibility variants in pediatric patients with eosinophilic esophagitis. J Allergy Clin Immunol 2017. https://doi.org/10.1016/j.jaci.2017.07.010.

22. Kanikowska A, Hryhorowicz S, Rychter AM, et al. Immunogenetic, molecular and microbiotic determinants of eosinophilic esophagitis and clinical practice-a new perspective of an old disease. Int J Mol Sci 2021;22(19):10830.

23. Hiremath G, Shilts MH, Boone HH, et al. The salivary microbiome is altered in children with eosinophilic esophagitis and correlates with disease activity. Clin Transl Gastroenterol 2019;10(6):e00039.

24. Busing JD, Buendia M, Choksi Y, et al. Microbiome in eosinophilic esophagitis-metagenomic, metatranscriptomic, and metabolomic changes: a systematic review. Front Physiol 2021;12:731034.

25. Hussain K, Letley DP, Greenaway AB, et al. Helicobacter pylori-Mediated Protection from Allergy Is Associated with IL-10-Secreting Peripheral Blood Regulatory T Cells. Front Immunol 2016;7:71.

26. Shah SC, Tepler A, Peek RM Jr, et al. Association Between Helicobacter pylori Exposure and Decreased Odds of Eosinophilic Esophagitis-A Systematic Review and Meta-analysis. Clin Gastroenterol Hepatol 2019;17(11):2185–2198 e3.

27. Doulberis M, Kountouras J, Rogler G. Reconsidering the "protective" hypothesis of Helicobacter pylori infection in eosinophilic esophagitis. Ann N Y Acad Sci 2020;1481(1):59–71.

28. Molina-Infante J, Gutierrez-Junquera C, Savarino E, et al. Helicobacter pylori infection does not protect against eosinophilic esophagitis: results from a large multicenter case-control study. Am J Gastroenterol 2018;113(7):972–9.

29. Dowling PJ, Neuhaus H, Polk BI. The role of the environment in eosinophilic esophagitis. Clin Rev Allergy Immunol 2019;57(3):330–9.

30. Parashette KR, Sarsani VK, Toh E, et al. Esophageal microbiome in healthy children and esophageal eosinophilia. J Pediatr Gastroenterol Nutr 2022. https://doi.org/10.1097/MPG.0000000000003413.

31. Johnson J, Dellon ES, McCoy AN, et al. Lack of association of the esophageal microbiome in adults with eosinophilic esophagitis compared with non-EoE controls. J Gastrointestin Liver Dis 2021;30(1):17–24.

32. Brusilovsky M, Bao R, Rochman M, et al. Host-Microbiota Interactions in the Esophagus During Homeostasis and Allergic Inflammation. Gastroenterology 2022;162(2):521–534 e8.

33. Benitez AJ, Hoffmann C, Muir AB, et al. Inflammation-associated microbiota in pediatric eosinophilic esophagitis. Microbiome 2015;3:23.

34. Hill DA, Grundmeier RW, Ramos M, et al. Eosinophilic esophagitis is a late manifestation of the allergic march. J Allergy Clin Immunol Pract 2018;6(5):1528–33.

35. Guajardo JR, Zegarra-Bustamante MA, Brooks EG. Does Aeroallergen Sensitization Cause or Contribute to Eosinophilic Esophagitis? Clin Rev Allergy Immunol 2018;55(1):65–9.

36. Mishra A, Hogan SP, Brandt EB, et al. An etiological role for aeroallergens and eosinophils in experimental esophagitis. J Clin Invest 2001;107(1):83–90.

37. Rayapudi M, Mavi P, Zhu X, et al. Indoor insect allergens are potent inducers of experimental eosinophilic esophagitis in mice. J Leukoc Biol 2010;88(2):337–46.

38. Akei HS, Mishra A, Blanchard C, et al. Epicutaneous antigen exposure primes for experimental eosinophilic esophagitis in mice. Gastroenterology 2005;129(3):985–94.

39. Wolf WA, Jerath MR, Dellon ES. De-novo onset of eosinophilic esophagitis after large volume allergen exposures. J Gastrointestin Liver Dis 2013;22(2):205–8.

40. Suto D, Murata K, Otake T, et al. Eosinophilic esophagitis induced by sublingual immunotherapy with cedar pollen: a case report. Asia Pac Allergy 2021;11(4):e44.

41. Miehlke S, Alpan O, Schröder S, et al. Induction of eosinophilic esophagitis by sublingual pollen immunotherapy. Case Rep Gastroenterol 2013;7(3):363–8.

42. Rokosz M, Bauer C, Schroeder S. Eosinophilic esophagitis induced by aeroallergen sublingual immunotherapy in an enteral feeding tube-dependent pediatric patient. Ann Allergy Asthma Immunol 2017;119(1):88–9.

43. Fujiwara Y, Tanaka F, Sawada A, et al. A case series of sublingual immunotherapy-induced eosinophilic esophagitis: stop or spit. Clin J Gastroenterol 2021;14(6):1607–11.

44. Jensen ET, Shah ND, Hoffman K, et al. Seasonal variation in detection of oeso-phageal eosinophilia and eosinophilic oesophagitis. Aliment Pharmacol Ther 2015;42(4):461–9.

45. Ram G, Lee J, Ott M, et al. Seasonal exacerbation of esophageal eosinophilia in children with eosinophilic esophagitis and allergic rhinitis. Ann Allergy Asthma Immunol 2015;115(3):224–8.e1.

46. Reed CC, Iglesia EGA, Commins SP, et al. Seasonal exacerbation of eosinophilic esophagitis histologic activity in adults and children implicates role of aeroaller-gens. Ann Allergy Asthma Immunol 2019;122(3):296–301.

47. Wang FY, Gupta SK, Fitzgerald JF. Is there a seasonal variation in the incidence or intensity of allergic eosinophilic esophagitis in newly diagnosed children? J Clin Gastroenterol 2007;41(5):451–3.

48. Ekre M, Tytor J, Bove M, et al. Retrospective chart review: seasonal variation in incidence of bolus impaction is maintained and statistically significant in sub-groups with atopy and eosinophilic esophagitis. Dis Esophagus 2020;33(6): doaa013.

49. Lucendo AJ, Arias Á, Redondo-González O, et al. Seasonal distribution of initial diagnosis and clinical recrudescence of eosinophilic esophagitis: a systematic review and meta-analysis. Allergy 2015;70(12):1640–50.

50. Letner D, Farris A, Khalili H, et al. Pollen-food allergy syndrome is a common allergic comorbidity in adults with eosinophilic esophagitis. Dis Esophagus 2018;31(2). https://doi.org/10.1093/dote/dox122.

51. Pesek RD, Rettiganti M, O'Brien E, et al. Effects of allergen sensitization on response to therapy in children with eosinophilic esophagitis. Ann Allergy Asthma Immunol 2017;119(2):177–83.

52. Ramirez RM, Jacobs RL. Eosinophilic esophagitis treated with immunotherapy to dust mites. J Allergy Clin Immunol 2013;132(2):503–4.

53. Iglesia EGA, Commins SP, Dellon ES. Complete remission of eosinophilic esoph-agitis with multi-aeroallergen subcutaneous immunotherapy: a case report. J Allergy Clin Immunol Pract 2021;9(6):2517–2519 e2.

54. Jensen ET, Kuhl JT, Martin LJ, et al. Prenatal, intrapartum, and postnatal factors are associated with pediatric eosinophilic esophagitis. J Allergy Clin Immunol 2018;141(1):214–22.

55. Biedermann L, Straumann A, Greuter T, et al. Eosinophilic esophagitis-established facts and new horizons. Semin Immunopathol 2021;43(3):319–35.

56. Lucendo AJ, Santander C, Savarino E, et al. EoE CONNECT, the European Reg-istry of Clinical, Environmental, and Genetic Determinants in Eosinophilic Esoph-agitis: rationale, design, and study protocol of a large-scale epidemiological study in Europe. Therap Adv Gastroenterol 2022;15. https://doi.org/10.1177/17562848221074204.

Climate Change Factors and the Aerobiology Effect

Andrew Rorie, MD

KEYWORDS

- Pollen • Climate change • Aerobiology • Thunderstorm asthma • Extreme weather
- Air pollution

KEY POINTS

- Climate change has a significant effect on aerobiology.
- Globally, pollen seasons are becoming longer and more abundant.
- Data suggest that air pollution may increase allergenicity of pollen.
- Thunderstorm asthma is associated with aeroallergen sensitization.

INTRODUCTION

An acceleration of global temperature increase has been observed since the mid-nineteenth century. There has been a clear association with the increasing temperature and an increase in greenhouse gases stemming from the Industrial Revolution. The primary gases generated by anthropogenic activities are carbon dioxide (CO_2), methane, nitrous oxide, and halogenated gases. Since the Industrial Revolution, the average atmospheric CO_2 concentration has increased from 280 parts per million (ppm) to current day more than 415 ppm which is a 45% increase.[1] Along with the increase in atmospheric CO_2 levels has been a tandem increase in global average surface temperature of 1°C.[2] More concerning, the rate of warming has accelerated with 7 of the 10 warmest years on recorded having occurred since 2014.[3] To date, climate change has resulted in higher global temperatures, rising sea levels, glacier recession, arctic ice thinning, dispersal of plant and animal geographic range, altered precipitation events, and longer and more abundant pollen seasons.[4] Combustible fossil fuels within our energy system are the largest single source of greenhouse gas emission.[5] As the Paris Agreement was negotiated by 196 parties in 2015, global strategies have been implemented to reduce greenhouse gases. In 2021, for the first-time, wind and solar energy generated over a tenth (10.3%) of global electricity. This is up from 4.6% when the Paris Agreement was originally adopted.[6] Unfortunately, even after CO_2 emissions, plateau or reduced surface air temperature will continue to rise for a century or more.[7,8]

Department of Medicine, Division of Allergy and Immunology, University of Nebraska Medical Center, 985990 Nebraska Medical Center, Omaha, NE 68198-5990, USA
E-mail address: arorie@unmc.edu

Immunol Allergy Clin N Am 42 (2022) 771–786
https://doi.org/10.1016/j.iac.2022.05.007
immunology.theclinics.com
0889-8561/22/© 2022 Elsevier Inc. All rights reserved.

One of the most significant consequences of climate change on human health could be the impact on aeroallergens.[9] Not only does pollution have direct health effects on the human population but also effects on plants and pollen production. Up to one-third of the US population has an underlying atopic process including allergic rhinitis, asthma, and atopic dermatitis.[10] The Global Initiative for Asthma estimates that asthma is one of the most common chronic diseases and effects 300 million people globally.[11] There has also been clear evidence that the prevalence of allergic disease has increased over the past 30 years, and there are several theories as to the etiology of this increase.[12,13] The three categories of pollen, which illicit allergic airway disease, are tree, grass, and weed pollen. The severity of pollen-induced symptoms is variable between individuals but the quantity of pollen grain exposure and the allergenicity of the pollen plays an important role.[7] As a result, climate change could lead to altered pollen exposure, sensitization, and symptoms.[7,9,14] Warmer temperatures associated with climate change leads to earlier pollination and longer and more abundant pollen seasons. Although increased CO_2 concentrations stimulate plant photosynthesis, increase water use efficiency, and alter phenology.[15–17] The net effect of a CO_2-rich environment is that plants grow faster and larger at maturity.[18,19] The objective of this article is to review recent worldwide reports related to the effects of climate change on aerobiology including pollination, production, allergenicity, and interplay with climate events.

CLIMATE CHANGE EFFECTS ON POLLINATION

Ragweed is a notorious instigator of hay fever symptoms and is one of the most abundant pollen producers throughout North America in the fall.[20] Reports have suggested that ragweed may be responsible for more seasonal allergic rhinitis than all other plants combined.[21] Pollen from the genus *Ambrosia* includes *Ambrosia artemisiifolia* (short ragweed), *Ambrosia trifida* (giant ragweed), *Ambrosia psilostachya* (western ragweed), and *Ambrosia bidentata* (lanceleaf ragweed).[22] The major allergen for ragweed is Amb a 1, and studies have shown ragweed grown in a CO_2-rich environment produces more of this major allergen.[23] Although ragweed has a long-standing presence in North American, it did not make its appearance in Europe until the beginning of the twentieth century. Its subsequent spread throughout the continent also serves as an example of climate change-driven expansion of plant species. Short ragweed (*A artemisiifolia*) was likely originally introduced in Europe due to commercial activities.[24] To date, there are only two primary centers of ragweed activity in Europe with one being in Hungary expanding north toward the Baltic and the other in northern Italy and southeast France.[25] It has been forecast that as the climate warms, ragweed will further expand throughout the continent. Recent published reports suggest that climate change-driven ragweed expansion will result in common allergic health problems throughout Europe, including areas where none currently exist.[26] To study the effects of climate change on ragweed, researchers grew plants from seed in climate-controlled greenhouses at ambient CO_2 levels (350 ppm) and double-ambient CO_2 conditions (700 ppm). They found that pollen production increased by 61% ($P = .005$) in the plants grown in higher atmospheric CO_2 conditions.[27] As a surrogate marker for climate change, Ziska and colleagues studied urban ragweed pollen production over a 2-year period. The urban environment is considered a heat island as daytime temperatures are about 1 to 7°F higher than outlying areas, whereas nighttime temperatures are 2 to 5°F higher.[28] They reported higher CO_2 concentrations (30%) and increased temperature in the urban setting, which was correlated with larger ragweed plant size, increased pollen production, and earlier pollen release.[29,30]

Next, a study by Ziska and colleagues investigated the length of ragweed season at varying latitudes in North America. There were a total of 10 different National Allergy Bureau (NAB) stations that had completed ragweed pollen counts dating back a minimum of 15 years. The range of latitudes of the varying stations range from Georgetown, Texas (latitude 30.63° N) to Saskatoon, and Canada (latitude 52.07° N). There was a statistically significant increase in the length of pollen season by as much as 13 to 27 days at latitudes above 44° N since 1995.[22] This finding was largely attributable to longer frost-free periods.

Numerous studies have also reported the effects of climate change on varying tree species. In Madrid pollen counts from 1979 to 2018 showed that several tree pollens (Quercus, Olea, Cupressaceae) in the geographic area had their highest recorded counts in the preceding 5 years. This increase in pollen was significantly correlated with increase in temperature. It was also reported that onset of pollen season was 4 to 31 days earlier depending on the pollen type studied.[31] A report from Zhang and colleagues observed airborne pollen data from six (NAB) pollen stations from 1994 to 2011. Each of these stations was geographically distinct and included the following locations: Fargo (North Dakota), College Station (Texas), Omaha (Nebraska), Pleasanton (California), Cherry Hill (New Jersey), and Newark (New Jersey). They showed during this 17-year period that birch and oak trees flowered 1 to 2 weeks earlier and both the annual mean and peak value of daily pollen concentrations increased by 13.6% to 248%.[32] The similar reports of climate change effect on birch pollen production have been reported in Switzerland, Finland, Denmark, and Germany.[33–35] The effect of the changing climate on oak pollen has also been reported across the world including Spain, Turkey, and Greece.[36–38] Additional studies have shown that when Pinaceae and Betulaceae have been grown in CO_2-rich environments, they have more biomass and exhibit more abundant pollen production.[39,40]

Several studies from Dr Levetin's group in Tulsa, Oklahoma, have analyzed Cupressaceae pollen dating back to 1987. These studies have demonstrated a significant increase over time of seasonal pollen index and peak pollen production.[41,42] Wang and colleagues[43] used satellite imagery to estimate that Juniperus woodlands have replaced 130,000 ha of Oklahoma grasslands from 1984 to 2010. There is a continued expansion of nearly 4800 ha per year which is near the size of Manhattan, New York. There has also been a continued expansion of juniper pollen throughout the upper Midwest. This expansion has likely been driven by climate change.[43] In the early 1990s, juniper pollen was not considered a major allergen in Kansas City (Missouri–Kansas). Up until approximately 2000, the total juniper pollen collected per year was less than 2,500, with a fairly rapid climb to greater than 20,000 per year in 2015.[44] The similar reports of increasing Cupressaceae pollen production and sensitization have also been observed in Japan.[45]

The term "grasses" is generally applied to species belonging of the Poaceae family.[46] Up to 20% of the global land surface area is covered by grasslands making it a common cause of pollinosis.[46,47] A recent study analyzed pollen data in northeast Europe dating back four decades and reported that of all five locations studied (Brussels, Belgium; De Haan, Belgium; Helmond, the Netherlands; Leiden, the Netherlands; and Luxembourg City, Luxembourg) the length of grass pollen season has increased. This being a result of grass pollen season beginning earlier as global temperatures have risen. Despite the longer grass pollen season, there has been a trend of decreasing annual pollen integral at each station.[48] There have been previous studies also reporting a decrease in total grass pollen production with speculation that it could be a result of urbanization or expansion of woodlands.[49–51] In contrast, researchers in Spain have reported an increase in grass pollen production from 1996 to 2010,[52] and a separate Spanish study showed longer grass pollen season, increased grass pollen production, and worsening grass pollen severity.[53] Thus, understanding the effect of climate change with grass pollen is difficult to determine based on current data as there are multiple metrological variables associated with increasing grass biomass and these are not all species specific. This paired with the variables of expanding urban centers, changes in land use, and agricultural practices among others make grass pollen a challenging model. Contrary to the above reports, Kurganskiy and colleagues[54] suggested that the severity of grass pollen season could be forecasted based on a combination of regional preseason meteorologic conditions, land surface models, and taking into account increasing atmospheric concentrations of CO_2 under climate change scenarios. Based on their modeling, it was predicted the severity of grass pollen season may increase by 60%.

Air Pollution and Altered Pollen Allergenicity

The appreciation for air pollution being detrimental to human health goes back to ancient times with the inhalation of volcanic fumes causing death. Later in the thirteenth century, the burning of coal in England was linked to respiratory ailments.[55] One of the most notable events occurred in England in 1952 when several thousand people died after several consecutive days of intense smog with SO_2 in excess of 2000 µg/d.[56,57] Since then, efforts have been made to replace coal burning as a primary source of heat/energy, which has reduced type I pollution defined by a predominance of SO_2 and dust. The central issue has now become type II pollution, which results from combustible petroleum products and the emissions of volatile organic compounds.[55] Although type I pollution has been correlated with inflammatory- and irritant-driven airway disorders, type II pollutants have been observed to modulate allergic processes.[58,59] This is further supported by the findings of increased atopy within the urban population.[60,61]

Environmental pollution has been shown to alter pollen allergenicity. Cortegano and colleagues studied the effects of air pollutants on the *Cupressaceae* family (*Cupressus, Juniperus, Chamaecyparis, Callitris, Thuja, and Libocedrus*). Pollen from *Cupressaceae* is an important contributor to allergic airway disease throughout the globe.[62] In the Cortegano study, pollen from *Cupressus arizonica* was collected from cypresses growing in high-pollution industrial areas and from low-pollution residential area. The pollen was then used to perform allergy skin prick testing on 75 subjects with known *C arizonica* allergy. It was reported the skin test wheal (mm) was significantly greater ($P < .001$) for pollen collected from high-polluted area compared with pollen from a low-polluted area.[63] This finding was further supported by radioallergosorbent test inhibition testing demonstrating pollen from the polluted area demonstrated five times the allergic activity compared with the pollen collected from the low-polluted area.[63] Additional studies have shown pollution and increased ozone levels result in increased pollen allergenicity with rye grass,[64] birch,[65] hornbeam,[66] and *Parietaria* ssp.[55]

CLIMATE CHANGE AND EXTREME WEATHER EVENTS

Climate change is also expected to drive more extreme climate-related events which may significantly impact allergic airway diseases. These extreme events include thunderstorms, tornadoes, hurricanes/typhoons, floods, droughts, wildfires, heat waves, and straight-line windstorms. In 2021, the publication of the Intergovernmental Panel on Climate Change Sixth Assessment Report refers to the increased frequency and/or intensity of extreme weather events as an "established fact" that they have been accelerated by human-driven climate change.[67] In 2021, there were 30 large scale extreme weather events worldwide resulting in over 3490 deaths and displacing more than 4.5 million people.[68] It is estimated that 19% of the world land surface is currently affected by drought.[69] Without a significant change in water and land management, the United Nations predicts "drought will be the next pandemic."[70] The drought on the Colorado River worsened in 2021 and remains on track to be the most severe in the last millennium.[71] This is not unique to North America as similar drought-related issues have occurred in Argentina, Brazil, Paraguay, Cameroon, and China among others.[72–77] The paradoxic relationship with spring precipitation promoting underbrush growth followed by extreme drought throughout the remainder of the year has continued to drive Western US wildfires. The 2021 Dixie fire to date was the second largest in the history of the state of California and even created its own weather system of storm clouds and lightning. The smoke generated was so immense it effected the East Coast some 3000 miles away. The 3 million hectares burned by wildfires in North America and Canada in 2021 was dwarfed by the 18 million hectares burned in Siberia.[78] Additional research is needed to understand how drought and wildfire affect pollen production, dispersal, and allergenicity.

Severe thunderstorms and tornadoes can be catastrophic. Over the past 25 years, they have accounted for more than one-third of weather events costing billions of dollars in damage and remediation efforts in the United States.[79] It has been reported that there are fewer days with tornados but more days with multiple tornados or "tornado outbreaks."[79] In addition, the length of tornado season seems to be expanding. It is difficult to trend the frequency of thunderstorms but there has been an increase in the number of hail days per year and windstorms (derechos) which are often associated with severe thunderstorms.[79] Multiple global climate models have been in agreement and project an increase in frequency and severity of severe thunderstorms throughout the mid-to-late twenty-first century.[80–84] The Midwest and southern Great Plains are to be the most effected throughout the United States and more so during the months of March, April, and May.[85] According to the National Oceanic and Atmospheric Administration, there are an estimated 16 million thunderstorms yearly and that number is set to rise.

Extreme weather events are a consequence of anthropometric climate change and rare will continue to increase in frequency. There is a paucity of literature on how these extreme weather events affect aeroallergens and thus studies are warranted to understand the potential implication in aerobiology. The most studied type of extreme weather event and its interaction with aerobiology and health is arguably thunderstorm asthma (TA).

THUNDERSTORM ASTHMA

There has been a growing fascination with the phenomenon of TA over the past decade. TA serves as an excellent model of how multiple factors associated with climate change and extreme weather can result in devastating health outcomes (**Fig. 1**). The first published report of what would later be termed TA occurred in Birmingham, United Kingdom, in 1983.[86] Following a July 6th thunderstorm, there was an observed 10fold increase in the asthma exacerbations requiring hospital admission. Since that sentinel report, there have been 27 acknowledged TA events around the world (**Table 1**). Most of these have been in Australia, whereas others have occurred in the United Kingdom, Europe, North America, China, and the Middle East. Although these occurrences are relatively rare in the literature, they are likely underreported. The deadliest TA event to date occurred in Melbourne, Australia, on

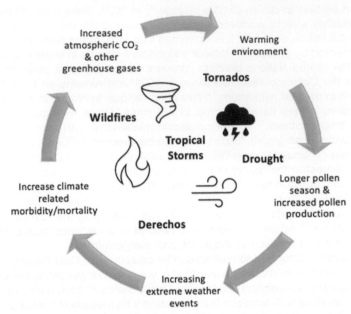

Fig. 1. Cycle of climate change and extreme weather.

November 21, 2016. During the 30 hours following the storm, the health care system was overwhelmed with a 672% increase in respiratory-related emergency room (ER) visits and 10 asthma-related fatalities.[87–89]

Owing to the tragic nature of the Melbourne event, more attention has been given to this phenomenon, but the environmental and immunologic mechanism of TA continues to be investigated. Most of the TA reports have suspected grass pollen as the trigger with more isolated reports of Mugwort, Olive tree, *Parietaria* pollen, and fungal spores.[90–94] There is a clear association in the Northern and Southern hemispheres with TA occurring during grass pollination season. Further evidence implicating grass pollen includes a study showing that 100% of patients who presented to the ED during the 2016 Melbourne TA event were sensitized to rye grass pollen (RGP). Furthermore, they had very high mean levels of antigen-specific IgE (sIgE) of 55 kUA/L (typical range <0.35–100 kUA/L).[95] It was also demonstrated that the rate of grass pollen sensitization was significantly greater in patients affected during the Melbourne event than unaffected severe asthma patients without grass pollen sensitization.[96] Similar findings have been reproduced by several groups.[88,97–100] Other pollen such as ragweed which is notorious for causing allergic airway disease has not been associated with TA. In the United States, over a quarter of the population is sensitized to ragweed.[101] A single ragweed plant can release 1 billion grains of pollen, although thunderstorms are relatively common during early ragweed season, there does not seem to be an association with TA.[102] The mounting evidence that TA events, particularly in Australia, are secondary to RGP sensitization has elicited further research into what makes RGP a unique aeroallergen in these events.

The most supported hypothesis of TA originates with high local pollen and/or fungal spore counts paired with an approaching storm front. Pasture grasses such as RGP are anemophilous (wind-pollinated) and a common global cause of allergic rhinitis.[46] The major allergen of RGP is Lol p 5, a prevalent spring allergen in Australia.[103] The

Table 1
Thunderstorm asthma events

Date	Location	Suspected Allergen	Reference
July 1983	Birmingham, United Kingdom	Fungal spores	Hughes and colleagues[115] 2020
June 1984	Nottingham, United Kingdom	Fungal spores	Alderman[94] 1986
November 1984	Melbourne, Australia	Not specified	Egan[116] 1985
November 1987	Melbourne, Australia	Grass pollen	D'Amato[117] 2020
July 1989	Leicester, United Kingdom	Fungal spores	[118]
November 1989	Melbourne, Australia	Grass pollen	D'Amato[117] 2020
November 1990	Tamworth, Australia	Grass pollen	Waters and colleagues[119] 1993
June 1994	London, United Kingdom	Grass pollen	Villeneuve[120] 2005
October 1997	Wagga, Australia	Grass pollen	Marks[121] 2007
October 1998	Newcastle, Australia	Grass pollen	D'Amato[122] 2008
July 2000	Calgary, Canada	Fungal spores	Allitt[123] 2000
July 2002	Cambridge, United Kingdom	Fungal spores	Suphioglu and colleagues[93] 1992
November 2002	Al-Khobar, Saudi Arabia	Not specified	Al-Rubaish[124] 2007
November 2003	Melbourne, Australia	Grass pollen	Bellomo and colleagues[99] 1992
June 2004	Naples, Italy	*Parietaria* pollen	Pulimood and colleagues[92] 2007
June 2005	South-East England, United Kingdom	Not specified	Levy[125] 2007
May 2010	Puglia, Italy	Olive tree pollen	Wardman[91] 2002
November 2010	Melbourne, Australia	Grass pollen	Marks[126] 2001
November 2011	Melbourne, Australia	Grass pollen	Marks[126] 2001
July 2013	London, United Kingdom	Not specified	Elliot and colleagues[127] 2014
November 2013	Ahvaz, Iran	Grass pollen	[103,128,129]
October 2014	Canberra, Australia	Grass pollen	C[130] 2014
October 2015	Israel	Not specified	Yair and colleagues[131] 2019, Rabiee[132]
October 2015	Ahvaz, Iran	Not specified	Rabiee[132] 2018
November 2016	Melbourne, Australia	Gras pollen	Thien and colleagues[88] 2018
December 2016	Kuwait, Middle East	Not specified	Ali and colleagues [133] 2019
December 2017	Hamilton, New Zealand	Not specified	Sabih and colleagues[134] 2020
September 2018	Yulin, China	Mugwort pollen	Xu and colleagues[90] 2021

Adapted from Thien F, Davies JM, Hew M, Douglass JA, O'Hehir RE. Thunderstorm asthma: an overview of mechanisms and management strategies. Expert Rev Clin Immunol. 2020;16(10):1005-1017.

intact RGP is approximately 30 μm in diameter making it a common cause of allergic rhinitis as pollen becomes lodged in the upper airway.[103] However, the intact RGP less commonly causes allergic bronchoconstriction because of the pollen size is considered too large to navigate the small airways.

On the leading edge of a thunderstorm, warm air masses cause updrafts which rapidly pull intact ground level pollen high into the atmosphere. Then, through a process of osmotic rupture and/or lightning/electrical rupture, the whole pollen grains are burst producing sub-pollen particles (SPPs).[104,105] Each grain can then release up to 700 starch granules (0.5–2.5 μm) which can more readily penetrate the lower airways leading to bronchospasm.[106,107] This may explain reports describing as few as 10% of affected patients in TA events had previously diagnosed asthma.[97] As the thunderstorm passes, the cold air mass on the backside leads to outflows or downdrafts which showers at risk individuals with allergenic SPP.

The major allergens of RGP Lol p 1 and Lol p 5 account for greater than 90% of IgE mediated symptoms in sensitized individuals.[108,109] Lol p 5 is primarily found in the starch granules, whereas Lol p 1 is found in the cytoplasm and secreted on the surface of the mature pollen.[110] When individuals experience symptoms of allergic rhinitis, it is typically the result of the presence of intact pollen in the upper airway and exposed to Lol p 1 on the pollen surface. During TA, the pollen grain is ruptured resulting in the release of SPP-rich starch granules and subsequent exposure to Lol p 5. After precipitation events in Melbourne, there was an approximate 50fold increase of these atmospheric starch granules reported.[110] Furthermore, Hew and colleagues compared 60 subjects who presented to the ER for respiratory symptoms during the 2016 Melbourne TA event to 19 control subjects with seasonal allergic rhinitis who were outdoors the day of the TA event but were asymptomatic. They reported there was no difference in sIgE sensitization to Lol p 1, but subjects that presented to the ER had higher levels of sIgE to Lol p 5.[103]

There is no current definition for what constitutes an epidemic TA event and capturing small, yet significant increases in asthma exacerbations after thunderstorms is challenging. For instance, the Nebraska Sandhills and Wyoming Basin are of the most intact seven largest grasslands on the planet.[111] These areas have the capability of producing massive amounts of pollen and the atmosphere of the Great Plains is ripe for supercell thunderstorm activity during grass pollination season. Yet, there are no reports of TA in these areas. Is this because TA is not occurring or is the population too sparse in those areas to appreciate a significant increase in respiratory events? Further evidence to suggest this phenomenon may be occurring more frequently than appreciated is a 10 year observational study in Atlanta, Georgia showing a significant increase ($P > .001$) of asthma-related ER visits on days with a thunderstorm.[112] Similar reports have been observed in Canada, United Kingdom, and Australia.[91,104,113] TA requires further research and there should be ample opportunity as TA events are projected to become more common.[114]

SUMMARY

One of the most readily demonstrated findings of climate change is the increase in CO_2 and the paired global increase in temperature. The interconnecting risks associated with climate change, extreme weather events, infectious disease transmission, and access to water will overburden the most vulnerable populations.[5] There are complex interactions between rising CO_2, increasing temperatures, and air pollution, but evidence strongly suggests there is a climate change-driven response of longer, more abundant pollen seasons and perhaps increased pollen allergenicity. These changes are likely to continue and forecast to worsen which will result in further morbidity and mortality of sensitized allergic airway disease individuals. In Australia, through diligent research much has been learned about TA. This has allowed for the development of TA early warning systems, improved public health awareness, and optimized asthma treatment for those at greatest risk. This serves as an excellent example of how the scientific community can work together to improve patient outcomes. Further research of the climate change effect on aerobiology is needed including associated health outcomes. As the world climate continues to change, the scientific community must continue to study and adapt.

CLINICS CARE POINTS

- Practitioners should educate patients with allergic airway disease to be aware of pollen counts and air quality.
- Patients at risk of thunderstorm asthma should have pre-seasonal asthma therapies optimized.
- Physicians should be familiar with environmental advocacy as it is a critical component of public health.
- Additional efforts are needed to develop accurate short-term pollen and fungal spore forecasting to prevent morbidity and mortality.

ACKNOWLEDGMENTS

The author thanks Dr Jill Poole M.D. (University of Nebraska Medical Center) for her comments on this article.

DISCLOSURE

"The author has nothing to disclose."

REFERENCES

1. Carbon dioixide peaks near 420 part per million at Mauna Loa observatory. NOAA Research News. Available at: https://research.noaa.gov/article/ArtMID/587/ArticleID/2764/Coronavirus-response-barely-slows-rising-carbon-dioxide, 2021. Accessed April 15, 2022.
2. Greenhouse gases. National Oceanic and Atmospheric Administration. Available at: https://www.ncdc.noaa.gov/monitoring-references/faq/greenhouse-gases.php. Accessed April 15, 2022.
3. More near-record warm years are likely on the horizon. . National Oceanic and Atmospheric Administration National Centers for Environmental Information. 2021. Available at: https://www.ncei.noaa.gov/news/projected-ranks. Accessed April 15, 2022.
4. Overview: weather, global warming and climate change. . National Aeronautics and Space Administration Global Climate Change. 2021. Available at: https://climate.nasa.gov/resources/global-warming-vs-cimate-change/. Accessed April 15, 2022.
5. Romanello M, McGushin A, Di Napoli C, et al. The 2021 report of the Lancet Countdown on health and climate change: code red for a healthy future. Lancet 2021;398(10311):1619–62.

6. D.J.. Global electricity review. 2021. Available at: https://ember-climate.org/insights/research/global-electricity-review-2022/. Accessed April 15, 2022.

7. D'Amato G, Holgate S, Pawankar R, et al. Meteorological conditions, climate change, new emerging factors, and asthma and related allergic disorders. A statement of the World Allergy Organization. World Allergy Organ J 2015; 8(1):25.

8. Watts N, Amann M, Arnelll N, et al. The 2018 report of the Lancet Countdown on health and climate change: shaping the health of nations for centuries to come. Lancet 2018;392(10163):2479–514.

9. Katelaris CH, Beggs PJ. Climate change: allergens and allergic diseases. Intern Med J 2018;48(2):129–34.

10. Demain JG. Climate Change and the Impact on Respiratory and Allergic Disease: 2018. Curr Allergy Asthma Rep 2018;18(4):22.

11. Available at: www.ginaasthma.org.2017. G.I.f.A.G, Accessed April 15, 2022.

12. Frenz DA. Interpreting atmospheric pollen counts for use in clinical allergy: allergic symptomology. Ann Allergy Asthma Immunol 2001;86(2):150–8.

13. Sly RM. Changing prevalence of allergic rhinitis and asthma. Ann Allergy Asthma Immunol 1999;82(3):233–48, quiz 248-52.

14. Annesi-Maesano I. United Nations Climate Change Conferences: COP21 a lost opportunity for asthma and allergies and preparing for COP22. J Allergy Clin Immunol 2016;138(1):57–8.

15. CURTIS PS. A meta-analysis of leaf gas exchange and nitrogen in trees grown under elevated carbon dioxide. Plant Cell Environ 1996;19(2):127–37.

16. Reekie JYC, Hicklenton PR, Reekie EG. Effects of elevated $CO2$ on time of flowering in four short-day and four long-day species. Can J Bot 1994;72(4):533–8.

17. Tyree MT, Alexander J. Plant water relations and the effects of elevated $CO2$: a review and suggestions for future research. Vegetation 1993;104(1):47–62.

18. Bazzaz FA. The Response of Natural Ecosystems to the Rising Global $CO2$ Levels. Annu Rev Ecol Syst 1990;21:167–96.

19. Curtis PS, Wang X. A meta-analysis of elevated $CO2$ effects on woody plant mass, form, and physiology. Oecologia 1998;113(3):299–313.

20. Lewis WH VP, Zenger VE. Airborne and allergenic pollen of north America. Baltimore, MD: Johns Hopkins University Press; 1983.

21. Wodehouse RP. *Hay Fever Plants*. 2nd ed. Hafner; 1971.

22. Ziska L, Knowlton K, Rogers C, et al. Recent warming by latitude associated with increased length of ragweed pollen season in central North America. Proc Natl Acad Sci U S A 2011;108(10):4248–51.

23. Singer BD, Ziska L, Frenz D, et al. Research note: Increasing Amb a 1 content in common ragweed (Ambrosia artemisiifolia) pollen as a function of rising atmospheric $CO2$ concentration. Funct Plant Biol 2005;32(7):667–70.

24. Hufnagel L, M L, Matyasovaszky I. The History of Ragweed in the World. Appl Ecol Environ Res 2015;13:489–512.

25. Berger U. Medical University of Vienna, D.o.O.-R.-L., Head of Research Unit Aerobiology and Pollen Information. Available at: https://www.pollenwarndienst.at.en.html. Accessed April 15, 2022.

26. Lake IR, Jones N, Agnew M, et al. Climate Change and Future Pollen Allergy in Europe. Environ Health Perspect 2017;125(3):385–91.

27. Wayne P, Foster S, Connolly J, et al. Production of allergenic pollen by ragweed (Ambrosia artemisiifolia L.) is increased in $CO2$-enriched atmospheres. Ann Allergy Asthma Immunol 2002;88(3):279–82.

28. Agency, U.S.E.P., Heat Islands. Available at: https://www.epa.gov/heatislands. Accessed April 15, 2022.
29. Ziska LH. Evaluation of the growth response of six invasive species to past, present and future atmospheric carbon dioxide. J Exp Bot 2003;54(381):395–404.
30. Ziska LH, Gebhard D, Frenz D, et al. Cities as harbingers of climate change: common ragweed, urbanization, and public health. J Allergy Clin Immunol 2003;111(2):290–5.
31. Subiza J, Cabrera M, Cardenas-Rebollo JM, et al. Influence of climate change on airborne pollen concentrations in Madrid, 1979-2018. Clin Exp Allergy 2022;52(4):574–7.
32. Zhang Y, Bielory L, Georgopoulos PG. Climate change effect on Betula (birch) and Quercus (oak) pollen seasons in the United States. Int J Biometeorol 2014; 58(5):909–19.
33. Estrella N MA, Kramer U, Behrendt H. Integration 289 of flowering dates in phenology and pollen counts in aerobiology: analysis of their spatial and temporal coherence in Germany. Int J Biometeorol 2006;51:49–59.
34. Frei T, Gassner E. Climate change and its impact on birch pollen quantities and the start of the pollen season an example from Switzerland for the period 1969-2006. Int J Biometeorol 2008;52(7):667–74.
35. Yli-Panula E, Fekedulegen D, Green B, et al. Analysis of airborne betula pollen in Finland; a 31-year perspective. Int J Environ Res Public Health 2009;6(6): 1706–23.
36. Damialis A HJ, Gioulekas D, Vokou D. Long-term trends in atmospheric pollen levels in the city of Thessaloniki, Greece. Atmos Environ 2007;41(33):7011–21.
37. Erkan PaBai Adem AM. Analysis of airborne pollen fall in Tkirdag, Turkey. Asthma Allergy Immunol 2010;8:46–54.
38. Garcia-Mozo H, Galan C, Jato V, et al. Quercus pollen season dynamics in the Iberian peninsula: response to meteorological parameters and possible consequences of climate change. Ann Agric Environ Med 2006;13(2):209–24.
39. LaDeau SL, Clark J. Pollen production by Pinus taeda growing in elevated atmospheric CO2. Funct Ecol 2006;20:541–7.
40. Darbah JN, Kubiske M, Nelson N, et al. Effects of decadal exposure to interacting elevated CO2 and/or O3 on paper birch (Betula papyrifera) reproduction. Environ Pollut 2008;155(3):446–52.
41. Howard LE, Levetin E. Ambrosia pollen in Tulsa, Oklahoma: aerobiology, trends, and forecasting model development. Ann Allergy Asthma Immunol 2014;113(6): 641–6.
42. Flonard M, Lo E, Levetin E. Increasing Juniperus virginiana L. pollen in the Tulsa atmosphere: long-term trends, variability, and influence of meteorological conditions. Int J Biometeorol 2018;62(2):229–41.
43. Wang J, Xiao X, Qin Y, et al. Characterizing the encroachment of juniper forests into sub-humid and semi-arid prairies from 1984 to 2010 using PALSAR and Landsat data. Remote Sensing Environ 2018;205:166–79.
44. Barnes CS. Impact of climate change on pollen and respiratory disease. Curr Allergy Asthma Rep 2018;18(11):59.
45. Kishikawa R, Koto E. Effect of climate change on allergenic airborne pollen in Japan. Immunol Allergy Clin N Am 2021;41(1):111–25.
46. Garcia-Mozo H. Poaceae pollen as the leading aeroallergen worldwide: A review. Allergy 2017;72(12):1849–58.
47. D'Amato G, Bonini C, Nunes C, et al. Allergenic pollen and pollen allergy in Europe. Allergy 2007;62(9):976–90.

48. de Weger LA, Bruffaerts N, Koenders M, et al. Long-term pollen monitoring in the benelux: evaluation of allergenic pollen levels and temporal variations of pollen seasons. Front Allergy 2021;2:676176.

49. Charalampopoulos A, Damialis A, Lazarina M, et al. Spatiotemporal assessment of airborne pollen in the urban environment: the pollenscape of Thessaloniki as a case study. Atmos Environ 2021;247:118185.

50. Rodríguez-Rajo F, Astray G, Ferreiro-Lage J, et al. Evaluation of atmospheric Poaceae pollen concentration using a neural network applied to a coastal Atlantic climate region. Neural Networks 2010;23(3):419–25.

51. Levetin E. Aeroallergens and climate change in tulsa, oklahoma: long-term trends in the south central United States. Front Allergy 2021;2:726445.

52. Garcia-Mozo H, Oteros JA, Galan C. Impact of land cover changes and climate on the main airborne pollen types in Southern Spain. Sci Total Environ 2016; 548-549:221–8.

53. García-Mozo H, Galan C, Alcazar P, et al. Trends in grass pollen season in southern Spain. Aerobiologia 2010;26(2):157–69.

54. Kurganskiy A, Creer S, de Vere N, et al. Predicting the severity of the grass pollen season and the effect of climate change in Northwest Europe. Sci Adv 2021; 7(13):eabd7658.

55. Bartra J, Mullol J, Davila I, et al. Air pollution and allergens. J Investig Allergol Clin Immunol 2007;17(Suppl 2):3–8.

56. Polivka BJ. The Great London Smog of 1952. Am J Nurs 2018;118(4):57–61.

57. Great Britain Ministry of Health. Mortality and morbidity during the London fog of December 1952. London: HMSO; 1954.

58. Behrendt H, Becker W, Fritzsche C, et al. Air pollution and allergy: experimental studies on modulation of allergen release from pollen by air pollutants. Int Arch Allergy Immunol 1997;113(1–3):69–74.

59. Ring J, Eberlein-Koenig B, Behrendt H. Environmental pollution and allergy. Ann Allergy Asthma Immunol 2001;87(6 Suppl 3):2–6.

60. Riedler J, Eder W, Oberfeld G, et al. Austrian children living on a farm have less hay fever, asthma and allergic sensitization. Clin Exp Allergy 2000;30(2): 194–200.

61. Nicolaou N, Siddique N, Custovic A. Allergic disease in urban and rural populations: increasing prevalence with increasing urbanization. Allergy 2005;60(11): 1357–60.

62. Bousquet J, Knani J, Hejjaoui A, et al. Heterogeneity of atopy. I. Clinical and immunologic characteristics of patients allergic to cypress pollen. Allergy 1993;48(3):183–8.

63. Cortegano I, Civantos E, Aceituno E, et al. Cloning and expression of a major allergen from Cupressus arizonica pollen, Cup a 3, a PR-5 protein expressed under polluted environment. Allergy 2004;59(5):485–90.

64. Eckl-Dorna J, Klein B, Reichenauer T, et al. Exposure of rye (Secale cereale) cultivars to elevated ozone levels increases the allergen content in pollen. J Allergy Clin Immunol 2010;126(6):1315–7.

65. Beck I, Jochner S, Giles S, et al. High environmental ozone levels lead to enhanced allergenicity of birch pollen. PLoS One 2013;8(11):e80147.

66. Cuinica LG, Abreu I, Esteves da Silva J. Effect of air pollutant NO(2) on Betula pendula, Ostrya carpinifolia and Carpinus betulus pollen fertility and human allergenicity. Environ Pollut 2014;186:50–5.

67. IPCCb. Weather and climate extreme events in a changing climate. . Intergovernmental Panel on climate change. 2021. Available at: https://www.ipcc.ch/report/ar6/wg1/#fullreport,2021. Accessed April 15, 2022.
68. Sheehan MC. 2021 Climate and health review - uncharted territory: extreme weather events and morbidity. Int J Health Serv 2022;52(2):189–200.
69. Rocque RJ, Beaudoin C, Ndjaboue R, et al. Health effects of climate change: an overview of systematic reviews. BMJ Open 2021;11(6):e046333.
70. UNDRR, GAR Special report on drought 2021. United Nations Disaster Risk Reduction. 2021. Available at: https://www.undrr.org/publication/gar-special-report-drought-2021. Accessed April 15, 2022.
71. Kann D, RR, Wolf D. The Southwest's most important river is drying up. CNN. 2021. Available at: https://www.cnn.com/interactive/2021/08/us/colorado-river-water-shortage/. Accessed April 15, 2022.
72. Yin Z, Wan Y, Zhang Y, et al. Why super sandstorm 2021 in North China? Natl Sci Rev 2022;9(3):nwab165.
73. BBC, South America's drought-hit Paraná river at a 77-year low. BBC. 1. 2021. Available at: https://www.bbc.com/news/world-latin-america-58408791. Accessed April 15, 2022.
74. W, C., Paraguay on the brink as historic drought depletes river, its life-giving artery. The Guardian. 2021. Available at: https://www.theguardian.com/global-development/2021/sep/27/paraguay-severe-drought-depletes-river. Accessed April 15, 2022.
75. Cimatti BV, TN. Cloud seeding and water rationing in drought-stricken Latin America. Wilson Center. 2021. Available at: https://www.wilsoncenter.org/blog-post/cloud-seeding-and-water-rationing-drought-stricken-latin-america. Accessed April 15, 2022.
76. VOA, Drought in Lake Chad region heightens conflicts between herders and farmers. Voice of America. 2021. Available at: https://www.voanews.com/a/drought-in-lake-chad-region-heightens-conflicts-between-herders-and-farmers/6358662.html. Accessed April 15, 2022.
77. AAS, Why super sandstorm 2021 in North China. American Association for the Advancement of Science, EurekAlert! 2021. Accessed April 15, 2022
78. A, R., Russia forest fire damage worst since records began, says greenpeace. The Guardian. 2021. Available at: https://www.theguardian.com/world/2021/sep/22/russia-forest-fire-damage-worst-since-records-began-says-greenpeace. Accessed April 15, 2022.
79. Program, U.S.G.C.R., Chapter 9: Extreme Storms. 2017. Available at: https://science2017.globalchange.gov/chapter/9/.
80. Gensini VA, Ramseyer C, Mote TL. Future convective environments using NARCCAP. Int J Climatology 2014;34(5):1699–705.
81. Seeley JT, Romps DM. The Effect of Global Warming on Severe Thunderstorms in the United States. J Clim 2015;28(6):2443–58.
82. Trapp RJ, Diffenbaugh N, Brooks H, et al. Changes in severe thunderstorm environment frequency during the 21st century caused by anthropogenically enhanced global radiative forcing. Proc Natl Acad Sci 2007;104(50):19719–23.
83. Van Klooster SL, Roebber PJ. Surface-Based Convective Potential in the Contiguous United States in a Business-as-Usual Future Climate. J Clim 2009;22(12):3317–30.
84. Del Genio AD, Yao M-S, Jonas J. Will moist convection be stronger in a warmer climate? Geophys Res Lett 2007;34(16):1–5.

85. Diffenbaugh NS, Scherer M, Trapp RJ. Robust increases in severe thunderstorm environments in response to greenhouse forcing. Proc Natl Acad Sci U S A 2013;110(41):16361–6.

86. Packe GE, Ayres JG. Asthma outbreak during a thunderstorm. Lancet 1985; 2(8448):199–204.

87. Hew M, Lee J, Nugroho H, et al. The 2016 Melbourne thunderstorm asthma epidemic: Risk factors for severe attacks requiring hospital admission. Allergy 2019;74(1):122–30.

88. Thien F, Beggs P, Csutoros D, et al. The Melbourne epidemic thunderstorm asthma event 2016: an investigation of environmental triggers, effect on health services, and patient risk factors. Lancet Planet Health 2018;2(6):e255–63.

89. Harun NS, Lachapelle P, Douglass J. Thunderstorm-triggered asthma: what we know so far. J Asthma Allergy 2019;12:101–8.

90. Xu YY, Xue T, Li HR, et al. Retrospective analysis of epidemic thunderstorm asthma in children in Yulin, northwest China. Pediatr Res 2021;89(4):958–61.

91. Wardman AE, Stefani D, MacDonald JC. Thunderstorm-associated asthma or shortness of breath epidemic: a Canadian case report. Can Respir J 2002; 9(4):267–70.

92. Pulimood TB, Corden J, Bryden C, et al. Epidemic asthma and the role of the fungal mold Alternaria alternata. J Allergy Clin Immunol 2007;120(3):610–7.

93. Suphioglu C, Singh M, Taylor P, et al. Mechanism of grass-pollen-induced asthma. Lancet 1992;339(8793):569–72.

94. Alderman PM, Sloan JP, Basran GS. Asthma and thunderstorms. Arch Emerg Med 1986;3(4):260–2.

95. Lee J, Kronborg C, O'Hehir R, et al. Who's at risk of thunderstorm asthma? The ryegrass pollen trifecta and lessons learnt from the Melbourne thunderstorm epidemic. Respir Med 2017;132:146–8.

96. Sutherland MF, Portelli E, Collins A, et al. Patients with thunderstorm asthma or severe asthma in Melbourne: a comparison. Med J Aust 2017;207(10):434–5.

97. Girgis ST, Marks G, Kolbe A, et al. Thunderstorm-associated asthma in an inland town in south-eastern Australia. Who is at risk? Eur Respir J 2000;16(1):3–8.

98. Howden ML, McDonald CF, Sutherland MF. Thunderstorm asthma–a timely reminder. Med J Aust 2011;195(9):512–3.

99. Bellomo R, Gigliotti P, Treloar A, et al. Two consecutive thunderstorm associated epidemics of asthma in the city of Melbourne. The possible role of rye grass pollen. Med J Aust 1992;156(12):834–7.

100. Erbas B, Akram M, Sharmage S, et al. The role of seasonal grass pollen on childhood asthma emergency department presentations. Clin Exp Allergy 2012;42(5):799–805.

101. Arbes SJ Jr, Gergen P, Elliott L, et al. Prevalences of positive skin test responses to 10 common allergens in the US population: results from the third National Health and Nutrition Examination Survey. J Allergy Clin Immunol 2005;116(2): 377–83.

102. Fumanal B, Chauvel B, Bretagnolle F. Estimation of pollen and seed production of common ragweed in France. Ann Agric Environ Med 2007;14(2):233–6.

103. Hew M, Lee J, Varese N, et al. Epidemic thunderstorm asthma susceptibility from sensitization to ryegrass (Lolium perenne) pollen and major allergen Lol p 5. Allergy 2020;75(9):2369–72.

104. Celenza A, Fothergill J, Kupek E, et al. Thunderstorm associated asthma: a detailed analysis of environmental factors. BMJ 1996;312(7031):604–7.

105. Emmerson KM, Silver J, Thatcher M, et al. Atmospheric modelling of grass pollen rupturing mechanisms for thunderstorm asthma prediction. PLoS One 2021; 16(4):e0249488.

106. D'Amato G, Vitale C, Lanza M, et al. Climate change, air pollution, and allergic respiratory diseases: an update. Curr Opin Allergy Clin Immunol 2016;16(5): 434–40.

107. Price D, Hughes K, Thien F, et al. Epidemic Thunderstorm Asthma: Lessons Learned from the Storm Down-Under. J Allergy Clin Immunol Pract 2021;9(4): 1510–5.

108. Ford SA, Baldo BA. A re-examination of ryegrass (Lolium perenne) pollen allergens. Int Arch Allergy Appl Immunol 1986;81(3):193–203.

109. Ong EK, Griffith IJ, Knox R, et al. Cloning of a cDNA encoding a group-V (group-IX) allergen isoform from rye-grass pollen that demonstrates specific antigenic immunoreactivity. Gene 1993;134(2):235–40.

110. Staff IA, Schappi G, Taylor PE. Localisation of allergens in ryegrass pollen and in airborne micronic particles. Protoplasma 1998;208:47–57.

111. Scholtz R, Twidwell D. The last continuous grasslands on Earth: Identification and conservation importance. Conservation Sci Pract 2022;4(3):e626.

112. Grundstein A, Sarnat S, Shepard M, et al. Thunderstorm associated asthma in Atlanta, Georgia. Thorax 2008;63(7):659–60.

113. Newson R, Strachan D, Archibald E, et al. Effect of thunderstorms and airborne grass pollen on the incidence of acute asthma in England, 1990-94. Thorax 1997;52(8):680–5.

114. Kevat A. Thunderstorm Asthma: Looking Back and Looking Forward. J Asthma Allergy 2020;13:293–9.

115. Hughes DD, Mampage C, Jones L, et al. Characterization of atmospheric pollen fragments during springtime thunderstorms. Environ Sci Technol Lett 2020;7(6): 409–14.

116. Egan P. Weather or not. Med J Aust 1985;142(5):330.

117. D'Amato G, Akdis C. Global warming, climate change, air pollution and allergies. European Journal of Allergy and Clinical Immunology 2020;75(9): 2158–60.

118. Literature review on thunderstorm asthma and its implications for public health advice. 2017. Queensland University of Technology for the Department of Health and Human Services. Available at: https://www2.health.vic.gov.au/about/publications/researchandreports/thunderstorm-asthma-literature-review-may-2107. Accessed April 15, 2022.

119. Waters J, et al. Epidemic asthma surveillance in the New England Region 1990-1992. N S W Public Health Bull 1993;4(9):100–1.

120. Villeneuve PJ, Leech J, Bourque D. Frequency of emergency room visits for childhood asthma in Ottawa, Canada: the role of weather. Int J Biometeorol 2005;50(1):48–56.

121. Marks GB, Bush RK. It's blowing in the wind: new insights into thunderstorm-related asthma. J Allergy Clin Immunol 2007;120(3):530–2.

122. D'Amato G, Cecchi L, Liccardi G. Thunderstorm-related asthma: not only grass pollen and spores. J Allergy Clin Immunol 2008;121(2):537–8.

123. Allitt U. Airborne fungal spores and the thunderstorm of 24 June 1994. Aerobiologia 2000;16(3):397–406.

124. Al-Rubaish AM. Thunderstorm-associated bronchial asthma: a forgotten but very present epidemic. J Fam Community Med 2007;14(2):47.

125. Levy M, Bryden C. Thunderstorm asthma. Br J Prim Care Nurs 2007;1:69–71.

126. Marks G, Colquhoun J, Koski M, et al. Thunderstorm outflows preceding epidemics of asthma during spring and summer. Thorax 2001;56(6):468–71.

127. Elliot A, Hughes H, Hughes T, et al. The impact of thunderstorm asthma on emergency department attendances across London during July 2013. Emerg Med J 2014;31(8):675–8.

128. Forouzan A, Masoumi K, Shoushtari M, et al. An overview of thunderstorm-associated asthma outbreak in southwest of Iran. J Environ Public Health 2014;2014.

129. Rad HD, Assarehzadegan M, Goudarzi G, et al. Do Conocarpus erectus airborne pollen grains exacerbate autumnal thunderstorm asthma attacks in Ahvaz, Iran? Atmos Environ 2019;213:311–25.

130. Colley Clare. Canberra sneezes through worst hay fever season in years. Canberra Times 2014.

131. Yair Y, Yair Y, Rubin B, et al. First reported case of thunderstorm asthma in Israel. Nat Hazards Earth Syst Sci 2019;19(12):2715–25.

132. Rabiee S, Mousavi H, Khafaie MA. Thunderstorm asthma outbreak, a rare phenomenon in southwest Iran: patients' perspectives. Environ Sci Pollut Res 2018; 25(36):36158–62.

133. Ali F, Behbehani N, Alomair N, et al. Fatal and near-fatal thunderstorm asthma epidemic in a desert country. Ann Thorac Med 2019;14(2):155.

134. Sabih A, Russell C, Chang CL. Thunderstorm-related asthma can occur in New Zealand. Respirology Case Rep 2020;8(7):e00655.

Electronic Cigarettes and Vaping in Allergic and Asthmatic Disease

Marissa Love, MD, Selina Gierer, DO*

KEYWORDS

- E-cig • Electronic nicotine delivery systems • ENDS • Vaping
- E-cig or vaping-associated lung injury • EVALI • Smoking cessation

KEY POINTS

- Vaping has become popular in many high-risk patient populations, including asthmatics and youth, both as an initial choice and an alternative to combustible cigarettes.
- The liquid used in vaping may cause adverse effects such as alterations in epithelial and sputum proteomes, airway gene expression, and mucus composition.
- E-cigarette (e-cig) or vaping product use-associated lung injury (EVALI) is a rare potentially severe and life-threatening acute or subacute illness often linked to vitamin E acetate.
- More information is needed about the long-term risks of vaping, specifically in high-risk patient populations like those who suffer from asthma and allergies.

INTRODUCTION

Electronic nicotine delivery systems (ENDS) such as e-cigarettes (e-cigs), vape pens, e-hookahs, e-pipes, tanks, mods, vapes, and other systems were introduced in 2006, offering alternatives to combustible cigarettes.[1,2] Their popularity is increasing due to stricter guidance on public smoking, advertising, discretion, and perception of a safer alternative to combustible cigarettes. There is significant controversy regarding their sale and regulation, particularly with youth. While also used for smoking cessation,[3] e-cigs have been cited as a gateway to drug use and subsequent use of combustible cigarettes.[4] They were deemed a "major public health concern" by the United States (US) Surgeon General in 2016.[5] Already associated with health consequences, recently e-cig or vaping product use-associated lung injury (EVALI) has exposed their potential to cause life-threatening complications.

This publication aims to educate readers on immediate and long-term health consequences of ENDS, so they may provide patient counseling on utilization focusing on the asthmatic population.

University of Kansas Medical Center, 3901 Rainbow Boulevard MS 2026, Kansas City, KS 66160, USA
* Corresponding author.
E-mail address: sgierer@kumc.edu

Immunol Allergy Clin N Am 42 (2022) 787–800
https://doi.org/10.1016/j.iac.2022.06.002
0889-8561/22/© 2022 Elsevier Inc. All rights reserved.
immunology.theclinics.com

SALES AND UTILIZATION

ENDS cornered the market by using product placement and reemploying advertising strategies used for traditional cigarettes banned in 1971.[6] Sales spiked from $6.4 million in 2011 to $2 billion in 2018.[5,7] Devices are relatively inexpensive and readily available.[1] With their small, discrete shape and lack of large vapor cloud, products such as JUUL are popular with youth and young adults, dominating the US market with nearly 70% of the sales.[8] "JUULing" has become a verb in popular culture. E-cig use surpassed traditional cigarettes in US youth in 2014.[5] Recent data on utilization:

- 4.2% of the surveyed adults currently using e-cigs were dual users.[5]
- 10.9% of surveyed US college students vaped tetrahydrocannabinol (THC) in 2018, up from 5.2% in 2017.[9]
- Estimated 5 million (27.8%) US high school students surveyed in 2019 used e-cigs, up from 20.8% in 2018% and 1.5% in 2011.[10,11]
- 11% of seventh grade students used e-cigs versus 6.8% used combustible cigarettes, and 42.2% had also used combustible cigarettes.[5]

Data from the National Youth Tobacco Survey revealed the common reasons youth began using ENDS (**Table 1**). One report found that 63% of surveyed JUUL users did not know that JUUL products always contain nicotine.[12] Evidence current e-cig users will evolve into dual users is mounting.[11]

Utilization in asthmatics is alarming, increasing from 20.3% (2014) to 29.1% (2017), most noticeable in those aged 18 to 24.[13] E-cig utilization may be more prevalent in asthmatic teens versus nonasthmatics as they report feeling less likely to become addicted and e-cigs were less harmful than cigarettes.[14–19]

Unfortunately, the data on increased utilization coupled with potentially at-risk populations highlights need to improve regulations, utilization screening, and patient counseling.

FEDERAL REGULATION AND WARNINGS

The Food and Drug Administration (FDA) Center for Tobacco Products regulates the manufacturing, importing, packaging, labeling, advertising, promotion, sale, and distribution of ENDS but does not have the ability to regular accessories. As of 2019, purchasers must be 21 by federal law.[20,21] Although often used for smoking cessation, they have not been approved by the FDA for this purpose due to lack of long-term use data and potential risk of EVALI and other potential serious lung disorders.[1]

DELIVERY DEVICES

Delivery systems include closed or open systems and tank or pod mods (**Fig. 1**). Open systems hold refillable e-liquid reservoirs enabling customization. Favored by youth with their discreet size and small vapor cloud, closed systems are concealable. Products are comprised of a mouthpiece, atomizer producing the aerosol from the liquid, battery (commonly rechargeable lithium), and sensor (**Fig. 2**). Powered e-cigs (brands:

Table 1 Reasons youth began using ENDS	
Use by a Family or Friend	39%
Availability of flavors	31%
Belief they are less harmful than other forms of tobacco (cigarettes)	17.1%

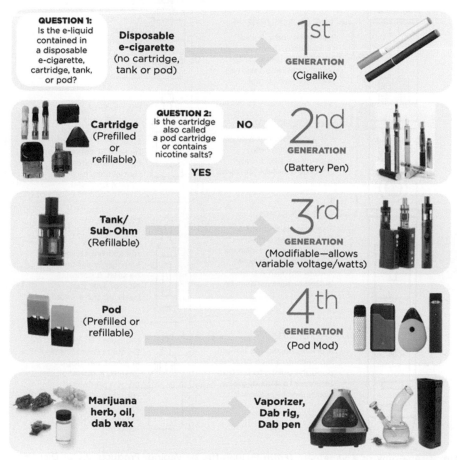

Fig. 1. Vaping product classification. (*From* E-cigarette, or Vaping, Products Visual Dictionary. Centers for Disease Control. Accessed April 28, 2022.https://www.cdc.gov/tobacco/basic_information/e-cigarettes/pdfs/ecigarette-or-vaping-products-visual-dictionary-508.pdf.)

JUUL, Bo, and myblu, and so forth) resemble USB devices, whereas disposables (brands: Zig Zag, Vapor4Life, V2, White Cloud, and so forth) are shaped like traditional cigarettes.[1] Vape peds (JUUL, Aspire, Apollo, Kanger, and so forth) feature discrete medium tanks.[1]

Tank mods have a customizable temperature, wattage, and nicotine (0–36 mg) delivery settings through their electronic control box (tank) along with refillable reservoirs. They are favored for smoking cessation to allow reducing nicotine exposure. Tank systems (brands: Aspire, Smok, Vaporesso, Kangertech, and so forth) may be disposable or rebuildable.[1]

Anatomy of an E-Cigarette

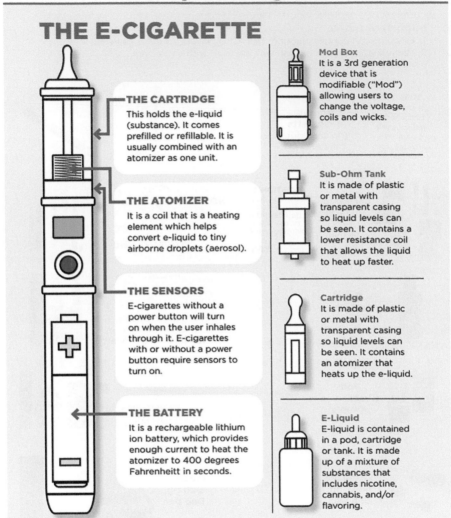

Fig. 2. Anatomy of a vape pen. (*From* E-cigarette, or Vaping, Products Visual Dictionary. Centers for Disease Control. Accessed April 28, 2022.https://www.cdc.gov/tobacco/basic_information/e-cigarettes/pdfs/ecigarette-or-vaping-products-visual-dictionary-508.pdf.)

Pod mods such as JUUL are inexpensive and feature discrete designs popular with youth and young adults. These products can deliver large amounts of nicotine disguised by flavorings unregulated by the FDA that have been proven to entice youth to begin experimentation with utilization.[12,22,23]

E-LIQUIDS

E-liquids and e-juices are flavor-filled inhalable aerosols that disguise the nicotine.[1] They contain flavoring, a solvent (vegetable oil/glycerin [VG] or propylene glycol [PG]), and varying quantities of nicotine. They turn into vapor by the heating element activated by a switch when the user inhales via the mouthpiece and the sensor detects a change in airflow, causing the battery to activate the atomizer to aerosolize the liquid. Depending on the product, a variety of chemicals may be found in the aerosols, many of which may be at toxic levels (**Box 1**).[8,24–27] Devices may also be used for vaping other products including THC, synthetic cannabinoid receptor agonists, crack cocaine, lysergic acid diethylamide (LSD), and methamphetamine.[28]

NICOTINE

Nicotine, a natural alkaloid component found at the highest concentrations in the leaves of the tobacco plant (*Nicotiana tabacum*), is a highly addictive stimulant.[29] Heating to decomposition emits nitrogen oxides, carbon monoxide, and highly toxic fumes.[30] Pharmacokinetics depend on the rate, location, and extent of absorption (**Table 2**). Nicotine is renally excreted (half-life of 1–3 hours) with more than 20 metabolites. While not pharmacologically active in humans, cotinine has a plasma half-life of 10 to 40 hours and may be used to assess for nicotine use in blood, hair, and urine.[31] The reported fatal adult dose is 40 to 60 mg or less than 5 mg/kg.[32,33] The nicotine delivery with ENDS varies between 3 and 36 mg/mL ranging up to 80 mg/mL.

Nicotine is an agonist of the nicotinic acetylcholine receptors, including those expressed in airways inhibiting cystic fibrosis transmembrane conductance regulator (CFRT) in airway epithelia.[29,34] It causes oropharyngeal mucosal inflammation, ulceration, altered taste, and skin irritation when applied topically. Dopamine release and binding of its receptors gives way to nicotine-induced euphoria and addiction.[31] Toxic effects include cardiac arrhythmia, vasoconstriction, hypertension, hyperglycemia, nausea/vomiting, abdominal pain, diarrhea, confusion, weakness, increased salivation and lacrimation, and respiratory alteration.[29,31] When delivered in a lower pH salt form, nicotine absorption is enhanced, and becomes less irritating.[35,36]

Tolerance and physical dependence may occur when smoking more than 100 to 150 mg of nicotine per day. Withdrawal symptoms vary, usually appearing within 24 hours of abstinence, and are characterized by behavioral changes, headache, and drowsiness.[31] Smoking while pregnant has been associated with increased risk of spontaneous abortion, low birth weight, and still birth.[32] Nicotine has been found to be a cocarcinogen in animals.[32]

FLAVORING ADDITIVES

There are greater than 7000 e-cig flavors including tobacco, menthol, fruit, candy, soda, and alcohol flavors commonly formed by ethyl maltol, ethyl vanillin, vanillin,

Box 1
Vaping aerosol contents
Organic Volatile Compounds: Propylene Glycol, Toluene, Glycerin
Aldehydes: formaldehyde, acetaldehyde, benzaldehyde
Acetone
Acrolein
Carcinogenic nitrosamines
Polycyclic aromatic hydrocarbons
Particulate matter
Metals: Chromium, cadmium, nickel, lead, copper, silver

| Table 2 | |
| Nicotine absorption | |
Product	Time to Peak Concentration
Intranasal spray	4–15 min
Chewing gum	25–30 min
Oral inhalation	15–30 min
Transdermal	2–10 h

cinnamaldehyde, and menthol. While typically considered safe for oral ingestion, there is limited evidence suggesting they are not safe when inhaled. In 2012, the Flavor and Extract Manufacturers Association of the United States identified priority flavoring agents with potential adverse lung effects including acetaldehyde, acetoin, benzaldehyde, diacetyl, cinnamaldehyde, and ethyl acetate.[37]

Flavoring agents can create toxic transformation products with aerosolization and heating. Aldehyde/formaldehyde and benzene formation, known carcinogens, occur primarily due to the aerosolization of flavoring compounds.[38,39] In vitro exposure to flavoring used in ENDS can be cytotoxic to human monocytes and has been found to trigger inflammation and oxidative stress.[40] Aromatic aldehydes (ie, cinnamaldehyde, benzaldehyde, and vanillin) impair neutrophil function.[41] Cinnamaldehyde caused a dose-dependent impairment in mitochondrial respiration and glycolysis, temporary reduction in adenosine triphosphate levels in human bronchial epithelial cells, and rapidly transiently suppressed ciliary beat frequency.[42]

PROPYLENE GLYCOL AND VEGETABLE GLYCERIN

In vitro and in vivo models demonstrate adverse changes in the airway due to PG and VG including airway remodeling, elevated MUC5AC in epithelial cell cultures, reduced membrane fluidity, and impaired protein diffusion.[43] PG and VG adversely airway epithelial cell viability.[44]

A pilot study of never smokers who underwent serial bronchoscopies after only PG and VG exposure revealed changes in BAL inflammatory cell counts and proinflammatory cytokines.[45] Contrary to their advertised inert biological behavior PG and VG may account for a significant portion of the airway damage in ENDS users.

PULMONARY COMPLICATIONS

Evidence is emerging on the detrimental health effects of ENDS, some resembling combustibles. ENDS devices use a variety of delivery systems, nicotine content, flavoring, and liquid compounds which can be customized, some products may be more detrimental than others.

In vitro airway models exposed to nicotine reveal macrophage activation[35] and impaired mucociliary clearance with altered epithelial cell surface liquid, mucous concentration, and mucous viscosity when exposed to e-cigs containing nicotine increasing the risk of infection and inflammation in the lungs (**Fig. 3**).[46]

Alterations in epithelial and sputum proteomes, airway gene expression, and mucous composition have been found with both combustibles and e-cigs. Changes in the aldehyde-detoxification and oxidative stress, immune suppression of host-defense genes; and elevation of MUC5AC, neutrophil elastase (NE), and matrix metalloproteinases (MMP)-2 and 9 have been found in allergic mouse airway samples (nasal scrape biopsies, nasal lavage, bronchoalveolar lavage [BAL], and induced sputum).[47]

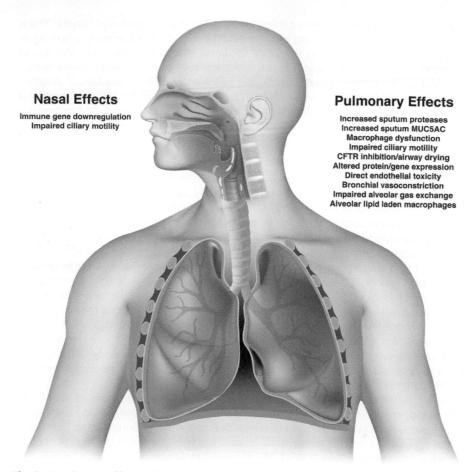

Nasal Effects

Immune gene downregulation
Impaired ciliary motility

Pulmonary Effects

Increased sputum proteases
Increased sputum MUC5AC
Macrophage dysfunction
Impaired ciliary motility
CFTR inhibition/airway drying
Altered protein/gene expression
Direct endothelial toxicity
Bronchial vasoconstriction
Impaired alveolar gas exchange
Alveolar lipid laden macrophages

Fig. 3. Respiratory effects of e-cigarettes.

MUC5AC elevation is implicated in increased airway obstruction and nonspecific airway hyperreactivity in asthma and COPD, while NE and MMP's have been implicated in tissue damage and remodeling. Additional mucus trafficking impairment with alteration in 113 proteins of epithelial cells causes concern for muco-obstructive disease.[43,48,49]

Riedel and colleagues also showed e-cigs alter the innate immune response leading to increased neutrophilic activation with elevated neutrophil-related myeloperoxidase and neutrophil extracellular trap (NET)-related proteins. These antimicrobial innate defense markers are associated with airway inflammation and damage, suggesting that e-cigs are not a healthier alternative for cigarette users. Additionally, their study showed that peripheral blood neutrophils isolated from e-cig users were more susceptible to NET formation compared with cigarette smokers and nonsmokers, which suggests the potential risk for harmful systemic disease.[49]

Immune gene suppression occurs in e-cig users versus nonsmokers, six times more than in cigarette smokers versus nonsmokers, concerning for increased risk of infection.[47]

Gross inspection on bronchoscopy of e-cig users reveals more friable and erythematous damage when compared with smokers and nonsmokers.[48]

Spirometry has been performed immediately after vaping with mixed results. There was no significant effect on lung function when comparing active e-cig smoking or having 1 hour of passive e-cig smoking.[50] A small study compared lung function in 10 healthy adult smokers and 10 nonsmokers after using a specific nicotine-free e-cig and showed only a small reduction in FEV1 and FEF25 in smokers.[51] Another study compared lung function in 20 healthy volunteers and 10 asthmatics after a one-hour vaping session and did not show any significant change in lung function using either spirometry or forced oscillation technique.[52]

ASTHMA

Although comprehensive and longitudinal studies regarding vaping are needed, asthmatics may be an at-risk population based on early data. Many e-cig aerosol chemicals are known respiratory sensitizers and irritants. Symptoms may include wheezing, which is commonly found in adolescents and adult e-cig users.[53,54] Asthmatics were found to have significantly increased airway irritation when compared with nonasthmatic smokers and recovery took twice as long after a single session of vaping using standardized settings but FeNo was decreased after a single session of vaping.[55] Among EVALI cases, common underlying comorbidity has not been clearly identified though 22% of the EVALI cases also reported a history of asthma.[56] There have been 2 case reports of life-threatening status asthmaticus requiring extracorporeal membrane oxygenation in teenage asthmatics.[56] Additionally, 1/3 of asthmatic teenagers were at increased risk of an asthma attack due to secondhand e-cig aerosol exposure.[57] Smokers with asthma were also more likely to have alterations in respiratory resistance following the single use of e-cigs as compared with healthy controls.[58]

There is a distinct emerging association between asthma symptoms as well as an asthma diagnosis in never smokers who use e-cigs.[59,60] E-cig use was independently associated with increased school absences due to asthma in South Korea.[61] In addition, e-cig use has been independently associated with asthma in US high schoolers (adjusted odds ratio = 1.48 [1.26–1.74]).[54]

E-CIGARETTE OR VAPING PRODUCT USE-ASSOCIATED LUNG INJURY

E-cigarette or vaping product use-associated lung injury (EVALI) is an acute or subacute respiratory illness that is potentially severe and life threatening. Imaging may be variable as are pathologic features. Though not the only cause, tetrahydrocannabinol products contaminated with vitamin E acetate were strongly linked to an EVALI outbreak in 2019 and vitamin E acetate was found in most of the bronchoalveolar lavage samples of patients with EVALI.[62] Vitamin E acetate, also known as tocopheryl acetate is a commonly used thickening agent for e-liquid containing THC. As of February 2020, there were roughly 2800 hospitalized EVALI cases or deaths reported to the CDC; however, cases have subsequently declined in the past 2 years.[63] Increased public health awareness, law enforcement, and removal of vitamin E acetate from products are thought to contribute to the decline. Proposed criteria for a confirmed case of EVALI include (1) use of an ENDS product in the previous 90 days, (2) lung opacities on chest radiograph or computed tomography, (3) exclusion of lung infection including viral infections such as influenza and SARS-CoV-2 and (4) absence of a likely alternative diagnosis such as cardiac, neoplastic, or rheumatologic processes. The optimal treatment of EVALI is not known but often includes antimicrobials until infection has been excluded as well as empirical use of corticosteroids.

12. Willett JG, Bennett M, Hair EC, et al. Recognition, use and perceptions of JUUL among youth and young adults. Tob Control 2019;28(1):115.

13. Desphpande M, Bromann S, Amoldi J. Electronic cigarette use among adults with asthma: 2014-2017 National Health Interview Survey. Res Social Adm Pharm 2020;16:202–7.

14. Fedele DA, Barnett TE, Dekevich D, et al. Prevalence of and believes about electronic cigarettes and hookah among high school students with asthma. Ann Epidemiol 2016;26:865–9.

15. Kim SY, Sim S, Choi HG. Active, passive, and electronic cigarette smoking is associated with asthma in adolescents. Sci Rep 2017;7:177–89.

16. Larsen K, Faulkner G, Boak A, et al. Looking beyond cigarettes: are Ontario adolescents with asthma less likely to smoke e-cigarettes, marijuana, waterpipes or tobacco cigarettes? Respir Med 2016;120:10–5.

17. Martinasek M, White R, Weldon C, et al. Perceptions of non-traditional tobacco products between asthmatic and non-asthmatic college students. J Asthma 2019;56:498–504.

18. Turner E, Fedele D, Thompson L, et al. Patterns of electronic cigarette use in youth with asthma: results from a nationally representative sample. Ann Allergy Asthma Immunol 2018;120:220–2.

19. McKelvey K, Bainocchi M, Halpern-Felsher B. Adolescents' and young adults' use and perceptions of pod-based electronic cigarettes. JAMA Netw Open 2018;1:e183535.

20. United States Food & Drug 2020. Newly Signed Legislation Raises Federal Minimum Age of Sale of Tobacco Products to 21. Available at: https://www.fda.gov/tobacco-products/ctp-newsroom/newly-signed-legislation-raises-federal-minimum-age-sale-tobacco-products-21. Accessed April 29 2022.

21. Centers for Disease Control. E-cigarette, or Vaping, Products Visual Dictionary. Available at: https://www.cdc.gov/tobacco/basic_information/e-cigarettes/pdfs/ecigarette-or-vaping-products-visual-dictionary-508.pdf. Page 15. Accessed April 28 2022.

22. Huang L, Baker H, Meernick C, et al. Impact of non-menthol flavors in tobacco products on perception and use among youth, young adults and adult: a systematic review. Tob Control 2017;26:709–19.

23. Rawlinson C, Martin S, Frosina J, et al. Chemical characterization of aerosols emitted by electronic cigarettes using thermal deportion-gas chromatopgraphy-time of flightmass spectrometry. J Chromatogr A 2017;1497:144–54.

24. Centers for Disease Control. E-cigarette, or Vaping, Products Visual Dictionary. Centers for Disease Control. E-cigarette, or Vaping, Products Visual Dictionary. Available at: https://www.cdc.gov/tobacco/basic_information/e-cigarettes/pdfs/ecigarette-or-vaping-products-visual-dictionary-508.pdf. Page 7. Accessed April 28 2022.

25. Lee M, LeBouf R, Son Y, et al. Nicotine, aerosol particles, carbonyls and volatile organic compounds in tobacco-and menthol-flavored e-cigarettes. Environ Health 2017;16(1):42.

26. Williams M, Bozhilov K, Ghai S, et al. Elements including metals in the atomizer and aerosol of disposable electronic cigarettes and electronic hookahs. PLoS One 2017;12(4):e0175430.

27. Goniewicz ML, Knysak J, Gawron M, et al. Levels of selected carcinogens and toxicants in vapour from electronic cigarettes. Tob Control 2014;23(2):133–9.

28. Blundell MS, Dargan PI, Wood DM. The dark cloud of recreational drugs and vaping. QJM 2018;111(3):145–8.

29. National Library of Medicine. Nicotine. Available at: https://pubchem.ncbi.nlm. nih.gov/compound/Nicotine. Accessed March 15 2022.

30. Lewis RJ Sr, editor. Sax's Dangerous Properties of Industrial materials. 11th Edition. Hoboken, NJ: Wiley-Interscience, Wiley & Sons, Inc.; 2004. p. 2636.

31. American Society of Health System Pharmacists; AHFS Drug Information 2009. American Society of Health-System Pharmacists: Bethesda, MD.

32. U.S. Environmental Protection Agency. Extremely Hazardous Substances (EHS) chemical Profiles and Emergency First Aid Guides. Washington, D.C.: U.S. Government Printing Office; 1998.

33. Zenz C, Dickerson O, Horvath E. Occupational Medicine. 3rd edition. St. Louis, MO: Mosby; 1994. p. 641.

34. Allen JG, Flanigan S, LeBlanc M, et al. Flavoring Chemicals in E-cigarettes: Diacetyl, 2,3-Pentanedione, and Acetoin in a Sample of 51 Products, Including Fruit-, Candy-, and Cocktail-Flavored. E-cigarettes Environ Health Perspect 2016;124(6):733–9.

35. Scott A, Lugg S, Aldridge K, et al. Pro-inflammatory effects of e-cigarette vapor condensate on human alveolar macrophages. Thorax 2018;73:1161–9.

36. Prochaska JJ, Benowitz NL. Current advances in research in treatment and recovery: nicotine addiction. Sci Adv 2019;5:eaay9763.

37. Angelini E, Camerini G, Diop M, et al. Respiratory Health – Exposure Measurements and Modeling in the Fragrance and Flavour Industry. PLoS One 2016; 11(2):e0148769.

38. Khlystov A, Samburova V. Flavoring Compounds Dominate Toxic Aldehyde Production during E-Cigarette Vaping. Environ Sci Technol 2016;50(23):13080–5.

39. Pankow JF, Kim K, McWhirter KJ, et al. Benzene formation in electronic cigarettes. PLoS One 2017;12(3):e0173055.

40. Muthumalage T, Prinz M, Ansah K, et al. Inflammatory and oxidative responses induced by exposure to commonly used e-cigarette flavoring chemicals and flavored e-liquids without nicotine. Front Physiol 2017;8:1130.

41. Hickman E, Herrera CA, Jaspers I. Common e-cigarette flavoring chemicals impair neutrophil phagocytosis and oxidative burst. Chem Res Toxicol 2019;32: 982–5.

42. Clapp P, Lavrich K, van Heusden C, et al. Cinnamaldehyde in flavored e-cigarette liquids temporarily suppresses bronchial epithelial cell ciliary motility by dysregulation of mitochondrial function. Am J Physiol Lung Cell Mol Physiol 2019;316: L470–86.

43. Ghosh A, Coakley R, Ghio A, et al. Chronic e-cigarette use increases neutrophil elastase and matrix metalloprotease levels in the lung. Am J Respir Crit Care Med 2019;200:1392–401.

44. Sossano MF, Davis ES, Keathing J, et al. Evaluation of e-liquid toxicity using an open-source high-throughput screening assay. Plos Biol 2018;16:e2003904.

45. Song MA, Reisinger SA, Freudenheim JL, et al. Effects of electronic cigarette constituents on the human lung: a pilot clinical trial. Cancer Prev Res (Phila) 2020;13:145–52.

46. Keismer M. Another warning sign: high nicotine content in electronic cigarettes disrupts mucociliary clearance, the essential defense mechanism of the lung. Am J Respir Crit Care Med 2019;200:1082–4.

47. Martin E, Clapp P, Rebuli M, et al. E-cigarette use results in suppression of immune and inflammatory response genes in nasal epithelial cells similar to cigarette smoke. Am J Physiol Lung Cell Mol Physiol 2016;311:L135–44.

48. Ghosh A, Coakley R, Mascenik T, et al. Chronic e-cigarette exposure alerts the human bronchial epithelial proteome. Am J Respir Crit Care Med 2018;198: 67–76.
49. Reidel B, Radicioni G, Clapp P, et al. E-cigarette use causes a unique innate immune response in the lung, involving increased neutrophilic activation and altered mucin secretion. Am J Respir Crit Care Med 2018;197:492–501.
50. Boulay M, Henry C, Bossé Y, et al. Acute effects of nicotine-free and flavour-free electronic cigarette use on lung functions in healthy and asthmatic individuals. Respir Res 2017;18(1):33.
51. Ferrari M, Zanasi A, Nardi E, et al. Short-term effects of a nicotine-free e-cigarette compared to a traditional cigarette in smokers and non-smokers. BMC Pulm Med 2015;15:120.
52. Vardavas CI, Anagnostopoulos N, Kougias M, et al. Short-term pulmonary effects of using an electronic cigarette: impact on respiratory flow resistance, impedance, and exhaled nitric oxide. Chest 2012;141(6):1400–6.
53. McConnell R, Barrington-Trimis J, Wang K, et al. Electronic cigarette use and respiratory symptoms in adolescents. Am J Respir Crit Care Med 2018;195:1043–9.
54. Schweitzer R, Wills T, Tam E, et al. E-cigarette use and asthma in a multiethnic sample of adolescents. Prev Med 2017;195:1043–9.
55. Laden JE, Ghinai I, Pray I, et al. Pulmonary illness related to e-cigarette use in Illinois and Wisconsin-preliminary report. N Engl J Med 2020;382:903–16.
56. Bradford L, Rebuli M, Ring B, et al. Danger in the vapor? ECMO for adolescents with status asthmaticus after vaping. J Asthma 2020;57:1168–72.
57. Bayly JE, Bernat D, Porter L, et al. Secondhand exposure to aerosols from electronic nicotine delivery systems and asthma exacerbations among youth with asthma. Chest 2019;155:88–93.
58. Lappas A, Tzortzi A, Konstantinidi E, et al. Short-term respiratory effects of e-cigarettes in healthy individuals and smokers with asthma. Respirology 2018;23: 291–7.
59. Perez M, Atuegwu N, Oncken C, et al. Association between electronic cigarette use and asthma in never-smokers. Ann Am Thorac Soc 2019;16:1453–6.
60. Li D, Sundar I, McIntosh S, et al. Association of smoking and electronic cigarette use with wheezing and related respiratory symptoms in adults: cross-sectional results from the Population Assessment of Tobacco and Health (PATH) study, wave 2. Tob Control 2020;29:140–7.
61. Cho JH, Paik SY. Association between electronic cigarette use and asthma among high school students in South Korea. PLoS One 2016;11:e0151022.
62. CDC. Outbreak of lung injury associated with the use of e-cigarette, or vaping, products. 2020. Available at: https://www.cdc.gov/tobacco/basic_information/e-cigarettes/severe-lung-disease.html. Accessed MArch 29 2022.
63. Smith M, Gotway M, Crotty Alexander L, et al. Vaping-related lung injury. Vichows Archiv 2021;478(1):81–8.
64. U.S Department of Health and Human Services. The health consequences of smoking-50 years of progress: a report of the Surgeon General. Atlanta, GA: U.S.: Department of Health and Human Services. Centers for Disease Control and Prevention. National Center for Chronic Disease Prevention and health Promotion, Office on Smoking and Health; 2014.
65. Berry KM, Reynolds LM, Collins JM, et al. E-cigarette initiation and associated changes in smoking cessation and reduction: the Population Assessment of Tobacco and Health Study, 2013-2015. Tob Control 2019;28(1):42–9.

66. Malas M, van der Tempel J, Schwartz R, et al. Electronic Cigarettes for Smoking Cessation: A Systematic Review. Nicotine Tob Res 2016;18(10):1926–36.
67. Hajek P, Pillips-Waller A, Przulj D, et al. A randomized trial of e-cigarettes versus nicotine-replacement therapy. N Engl J Med 2019;380:629–37.
68. Polosa R, Morjaria J, Caponnetto P, et al. Effect of smoking abstinence and reduction in asthmatic smokers switching to electronic cigarettes: evidence for harm reversal. Int J Environ Res Public Health 2014;11:4956–77.
69. Polosa R, Morjaria JB, Caponneto P, et al. Evidence for harm reduction in COPD smokers who switch to electronic cigarettes. Respir Res 2016;17:166.
70. Polosa R, Morjaraia J, Caponnetto P, et al. Persisting long term benefits of smoking abstinence and reduction in asthmatic smokers who have switched to electronic cigarettes. Discov Med 2016;21:99–108.
71. Farsalinos K, Romagna G, Tsiapras D, et al. Characteristics, perceived side effects and benefits of electronic cigarette use: a worldwide survey of more than 19,000 consumers. Int J Environ Res Public Health 2014;11:4356–73.

Air Pollution Effects in Allergies and Asthma

Anil Nanda, MD[a], Syed Shahzad Mustafa, MD[a,b], Maria Castillo, MD[a,c], Jonathan A. Bernstein, MD[d],*

KEYWORDS

- Air pollution • Urbanization • Epithelial barriers • Alarmins • Asthma
- Allergic rhinitis • Health effects

KEY POINTS

- Outdoor air pollution is associated with exacerbations of allergic diseases, including asthma, allergic rhinitis, and other atopic conditions.
- The main greenhouse gasses generated by human activity that cause health effects are carbon dioxide (CO_2), methane (CH_4), nitrous oxide (N_2O), ambient particulate matter, and gaseous pollutants including nitrogen dioxide (NO_2), sulfur dioxide (SO_2), and ozone (O_3).
- Air pollution and climate changes have led to increased geographic distribution of pollen, prolonged pollination seasons, and these higher pollen counts have contributed to health effects in allergic rhinitis and asthma sufferers; indoor and outdoor air pollutants act synergistically with allergens to magnify allergic responses.
- The epithelium functions as a protective barrier for many organ systems and disruption leads to a permeable epithelium causing dysbiosis, an imbalance in the microflora that can induce tissue inflammation.
- Changes in the microbiome are now recognized as being important for shaping the immune system and tissue homeostasis of the upper and lower respiratory tracts and gastrointestinal tract.

INTRODUCTION

Outdoor air pollution is associated with exacerbations of allergic diseases, including asthma, allergic rhinitis (AR), and other atopic conditions.[1] Both new onset of these conditions and exacerbation of existing allergic disorders have been shown to occur

[a] Division of Allergy and Immunology, Asthma and Allergy Center, Lewisville and Flower Mound, Texas, University of Texas Southwestern Medical Center, Dallas, TX, USA; [b] Rochester Regional Health, University of Rochester School of Medicine and Dentistry, 222 Alexander St. Rochester, NY 14607, USA; [c] Driscoll Children's Hospital, South Texas, USA; [d] Department of Internal Medicine, Division of Rheumatology, Allergy and Immunology, University of Cincinnati College of Medicine, 231 Albert Sabin Way, ML#563, Cincinnati, OH 45267-0563, USA
* Corresponding author.
E-mail address: bernstja@ucmail.uc.edu

Immunol Allergy Clin N Am 42 (2022) 801–815
https://doi.org/10.1016/j.iac.2022.06.004
0889-8561/22/© 2022 Elsevier Inc. All rights reserved.

with air pollution.[1] Pollution includes particulate matter (PM), gaseous pollutants (including ozone [O_3], nitrogen dioxide, and sulfur dioxide [SO_2]), and traffic related air pollution (TRAP).[1] PM (either PM_{10} [diameter: <10 um] or PM_5 [diameter: <2 um]) includes metals, such as copper, magnesium, zinc, and iron, which increase free radicals and reduce antioxidants.[2] This leads to a discharge of inflammatory cytokines, oxidative stress, and cellular damage.[2] Urbanization is thought to contribute to air pollution.[1] The increased allergic disease prevalence has been linked to this urbanization, industrialization, and economic growth globally.[3] This causes serious morbidity in allergic diseases.[4] This review provides an overview of the health effects of air pollution on allergic disorders and specifically addresses how it may impact the epithelial barrier in the upper and lower respiratory tracts to facilitate the health effects associated with these exposures.

AIR POLLUTION EFFECTS ON AEROBIOLOGY

Nearly 100 years ago, F. C. Meier coined the term aerobiology to describe a project evaluating the study of life in the air. Since that time, although there are various definitions, aerobiology is accepted as a branch of science studying the occurrence and effects of airborne microorganisms such as pollutants, viruses, and pollens. Regardless of the specific definition, the importance of aerobiology has become widely accepted to play an integral role in all aspects of human society, including space exploration, biological warfare, industrial as well as agricultural engineering, and human health.

The main greenhouse gasses generated by human activity are carbon dioxide (CO_2), methane (CH_4), nitrous oxide (N_2O). In addition, ambient PM and gaseous pollutants including nitrogen dioxide, sulfur dioxide (SO_2), and ozone have caused great health concerns.[5] Since the industrial revolution, the concentration of CO_2 in the atmosphere has increased by nearly 50%, from an average of 280 ppm to more than 415 ppm.[6] This increase in greenhouse gasses has led to increased global temperatures and has been a driving factor behind climate change, defined by the United Nations Framework Convention on Climate Change as "a change of climate which is attributed directly or indirectly to human activity that alters the composition of the global atmosphere and which is in addition to natural climate variability observed over comparable period."[7] Consequently, the increased production of greenhouse gasses has contributed to air pollution and decreased air quality. The World Health Organization reports that greater than 90% of the world's population live in areas of low air quality, where the concentration of pollutants exceeds recommended guidelines.[8] Air pollution is felt to be one of the leading causes of premature death around the world, with pervasive effects on human health affecting all body systems.[8] Although chronic obstructive pulmonary disease is the leading cause to death attributed to air pollution, air pollution affects non-respiratory organs as well and has a myriad of impacts ranging from mental health to ischemic heart disease.[9] Air pollution has also been linked to increased susceptibility to respiratory viral infections.[10] Potential mechanisms include changes in epithelial cell permeability and impaired local antiviral immunity by the imbalance of mucosal adhesion molecules and T-helper cells.[11] The importance of effects on respiratory viral immunity has never been more important than during the ongoing global coronavirus-19 (COVID-19) pandemic. Studies have suggested exposure to increased air pollution may increase frequency and severity of COVID-19 infection, potentially even contributing to mortality.[12] Finally, aerobiology has an undeniable impact on chronic rhinitis and asthma, reviewed in greater detail in subsequent sections of this review.[13]

Air pollution and changes in climate also have several indirect consequences that impact human health. Warmer temperatures lead not only to increased geographic distribution of pollen but also to prolonged pollination seasons, potentially starting a week earlier and lasting a week longer than previous decades.[14] Plants may also produce higher pollen counts, with increased allergenicity. Ragweed, for example, has been shown to grow faster in urban areas as compared with rural areas.[15] Similarly, birch trees exposed to more ozone produce more pollen as compared with trees in areas of better air quality.[16] Along with increased amounts, pollen adjacent to heavy traffic released more allergenic mediators as well, potentially leading to more significant symptomatology in atopic individuals.[17] Given that pollen not only carries allergen but also highly active lipid mediators (pollen-associated lipid mediators), exposure has immunomodulating effects, including increased local airway inflammation.[18,19] Even local events, like the attacks on the World Trade Centers in 2001, can impact aerobiology by changing local conditions. Following these attacks, there was increased O_3 and SO_2 in the New York City area, and this correlated with increased asthma-related emergency department visits.[20] Climate change also contributes to extreme weather events, such as increase hurricanes and cyclones, wildfires, droughts, and dust storms. In addition to obvious societal impact, these changes can also impact aerobiology in less obvious ways and can even alter indoor environments. Extreme weather can lead to widespread flooding, as evidenced by Hurricane Katrina in New Orleans and Hurricane Harvey in Houston. Flooding can change indoor conditions, leading to increased microbial and mold growth, and thus impacting sinopulmonary conditions. The indoor environment is also affected by several other factors, including surrounding outdoor pollutants and the quality and ventilation. Indoor activities such as smoking, heating, and cooking also impact indoor aerobiology.[21]

Although everyone is affected by aerobiology and changes due to climate change, there are certain vulnerable populations more impacted by this phenomenon. The impact can start as early as the prenatal stage and may impact children even more than adults. Prenatal exposure to air pollution is consistently linked to the increased risk of asthma and wheezing in children.[22] A meta-analysis looking at 35 studies across 12 countries on the impact of air pollution and AR found children and adolescents to be more susceptible as compared with adult counterparts.[23] At the other end of the spectrum, the growing elderly population may be similarly susceptible to changes in aerobiology. Individuals in urban centers also seem to be at a higher risk of disease as compared with those in more rural environments with increased green space. This distribution may also impact health care disparities and thus warrants special attention.

Given the noteworthy changes in aerobiology and its impact on human health, the question becomes on how to intervene in hopes of changing the current trajectory. Given the recent increasing rates of global warming, climate experts predict continued worsening of annual warming rates unless we implement aggressive mitigation strategies. On a microlevel, individual actions are necessary to affect change. In addition to raising awareness, strategies such as shared transport rather than individual transport can decrease emissions. Decreasing livestock produced by less reliance on meat consumption can impact CO_2 production. On a public health level, fossil fuels must be replaced by renewal energy sources. Without these policy changes, there will continue to be an irreversible negative impact on the planet and human health.

HEALTH EFFECTS OF AIR POLLUTION ON CHRONIC RHINITIS

Air pollutants can be classified as indoor or outdoor, primary (if they are emitted directly into the atmosphere), or secondary (if they react or interact with it, eg, ozone).

In this sense, biological air pollution is caused in part by aeroallergens that may preferentially contribute to atopic diseases indoors or outdoors, such as AR and asthma. AR is an Immunoglobulin E (IgE)-mediated type 1 hypersensitivity disease, triggered by a spectrum of environmental allergens such as outdoor pollen or mold spore allergens and/or indoor allergens such as dust mites, cockroaches, pet allergens, or molds. However, there are other rhinitis phenotypes such as vasomotor rhinitis that are not IgE-mediated but rather induced through neurogenic pathways, which are triggered by a spectrum of chemical irritants, odorants, or weather changes (ie, temperature, barometric pressure).[24]

Presently, the prevalence of AR induced by environmental pollutants in children and adults is poorly elucidated. Reasons for this gap in knowledge may be due to differences in epidemiological study design and exposure assessment methods including exposure duration.[25] However, most studies have found a strong interaction between air pollutants and AR.[26–28] A recent systematic review and meta-analysis found that the effect of air pollutants on AR, except for PM_{10}, was significant and higher in developing countries than in developed countries.[23]

Outdoor Air Pollution

The main outdoor air pollutants that affect health, such as particulate matter (PM), O_3, TRAP, and DEP, exist in solid or liquid forms and can be anthropogenic or naturally occurring during dust storms, forest fires, or to a lesser extent during volcanic eruptions.[29,30] Likewise, PM can vary in its composition[31] and size[32] and it has been shown in both in vivo and in vitro studies that fine and ultrafine particles are the pollutants most commonly associated with the pathologic changes that occur in the upper and lower respiratory tracts causing symptoms.[33]

In a multicenter study, in five European birth cohorts, it was shown that exposure to PM and nitrogen oxides was associated with a deficit in school-age children's lung function. This same association was also found in a study of five European adult cohorts which demonstrated that greater exposure to nitrogen monoxide (NO), NO_2, and PM_{10} from traffic was associated with decreased lung function.[34]

Although studies reporting on the relationship between rhinitis and outdoor air pollution continues to be inconsistent in both adults[35] and children[36]; it has been seen that people living in urban areas are affected more so than those living in rural areas.[37] In addition to the air pollutants already mentioned, there are other particulates related to the deterioration of respiratory health, such as livestock emissions such as organic dust, toxins from microorganisms, and ammonia or methane gases. For example, a Dutch study showed an association between high levels of outdoor air pollution and decreased lung function in rural dwellers including non-farmers.[38]

Indoor Air Pollution

A common source of indoor air pollution is tobacco smoke, which contains at least 4500 toxic chemical compounds, including PM, oxidizing gases, heavy metals, and at least 50 carcinogens. Recently, pyrosynthesis and cigarette combustion related to domestic smoking were identified as key phenomena that increase the levels of PM and toxic chemicals in homes.[39] In addition, other indoor air pollutants include nitrogen dioxide, carbon monoxide (CO), formaldehyde,[40] and chemical volatile organic compounds (cVOCs) such as those generated by construction materials or cleaning products. Generally, indoor pollutants are most frequently generated by gas cooking and heating appliances. Studies have found that the presence of indoor NO_2 increases or worsens asthma symptoms in children.[41,42] Similarly, a systematic review reported the existence of a weak relationship between cVOCs generated by building materials and/or cleaning products with AR, both in children and adults.[43]

An interaction between air pollutants resulting from the consumption of solid fuels, such as coal, and tobacco smoke exposure has been established for asthma in both adults and children.[44] However, until now, there is no conclusive evidence linking the different contaminating agents with AR. Similarly, an interaction between air pollutants and allergens such as mold, dust mites, and furry pets can exacerbate lower respiratory symptoms and reduce lung function,[45] but evidence for this effect on AR is weak and inconsistent.

It is important to emphasize that indoor allergens interact with air pollutants to generate more severe allergy phenotypes in the upper and lower respiratory tract compared with outdoor seasonal allergens.[46] In addition, the presence of humidity in homes or closed spaces can promote colonization of molds or cockroaches, resulting in allergen sensitization of inhabitants.[47,48] In addition, indoor mold infestation can trigger inflammation of the upper and lower respiratory tract through the production of microbial volatile organic compounds (VOCs) and less commonly through by-products such as beta-glucans or mycotoxins.

It has also been shown that both external and internal air pollutants act synergistically with allergen to magnify allergic responses. For example, one study showed an increase or amplification of allergic inflammation resulting from the inhalation of DEP before exposure to allergens in the lower respiratory tract of atopic individuals. This phenomenon may be due to the increased recruitment of neutrophils and eosinophils, resulting in the production of interleukin (IL)-8 and IL-5 cytokine production, respectively, as well as other inflammatory biomarkers such as eosinophil cationic protein and monocyte chemotactic protein-1.[25,49] In another study, it was shown that controlled exposure to ozone or VOCs in the upper respiratory tract of healthy individuals generates recruitment of neutrophils, suggesting the establishment of a Th1-type immune response pattern. However, ozone exposure in the lungs of both healthy and allergic patients generated increased recruitment of both eosinophils and neutrophils, suggesting the establishment of a mixed response pattern (T helper lymphocyte 1 [TH 1] and T helper lymphocyte 2 [TH2]) for this air pollutant. Finally, evidence suggests that DEP exposure biases toward a Th2 immune response pattern.[50,51] Collectively, these studies suggest that the establishment of the immune response after exposure to air pollutants varies depending on the subject population studied, their socioeconomic status, the respiratory organ affected, and the specific pollutant studied. It is for these reasons that data establishing a relationship between AR and air pollution are variable and often inconsistent.

HEALTH EFFECTS OF AIR POLLUTANTS ON ASTHMA

Exposure to air pollution has been associated with increased asthma mortality risk.[52] Outdoor air pollution at higher concentrations has a direct inflammatory and irritant effect on airway epithelium and at lower concentrations causes both airway hyperresponsiveness and inflammation, both characteristics of asthma.[1] The mechanisms include airway remodeling, oxidative damage, airway remodeling, the induction of immune responses, and increasing sensitization to aeroallergens.[1] Certain genotypes can enhance allergic responses to outdoor air pollutants, such as diesel exhaust particles.[53]

Airway pollutants and atmospheric agents involved with asthma include ozone, sulfur dioxide (SO_2), and nitrogen oxides.[54] In the United States, pollution sources such as power plants and other nonmobile industries are responsible for about 93% of SO_2

emissions, 51% of nitrogen oxide emissions, and about 52% of VOC emissions.[54] Mobile sources of pollution such as automobiles also contribute to these pollutants.[54] Ozone is produced from reactions in the atmosphere involving VOC, nitrogen oxide, and ultraviolet light.[54]

Ozone

Ozone causes neutrophil incursion into the airway, usually a few hours after exposure.[54] There is also eosinophilic inflammation associated with ozone exposure.[54] Other inflammatory mediators include IL-8, IL-6, leukotriene B_4, plasminogen activator, and elastase.[54] Epidemiology studies have shown increased emergency department and hospital admissions for asthma after increased atmosphere ozone concentrations, including between 160 and 400 ppb.[55] One large study demonstrated that an increase in ozone by 10 ppb resulted in an elevated risk of death from respiratory causes.[56] There is also a report of an association between fatal asthma and ozone in New York City.[57,58]

Sulfur Dioxide

Sulfur dioxide is associated with coal energy production.[1] In developed countries, levels have been lowered, but this exposure is still elevated in developing nations.[1] One analysis of multiple studies showed that exposure to sulfur dioxide increased risk of asthma exacerbations.[59] Sulfur dioxide has been associated with exercise-induced asthma also, leading to a decrease in Forced expiratory volume (FEV_1) by 23%.[58,60]

Nitrogen Oxide

Nitrogen oxides (including NO_2) are associated with automobile traffic.[54,60] There is evidence of a bronchoconstrictor response in asthma patients on exposure to NO_2 concentrations of 0.1 ppm.[60] In addition, bronchial hyperresponsiveness has been increased with NO_2 exposure.[58] Nitric oxide has also been associated with an increased risk of asthma exacerbations.[59]

Particulate matter

PM consists of multiple substances, including black carbon, metals, biologic contaminants, and organic residues.[54] They can include roadway dust, automobile tire wear particles, and automobile brake wear particles, and diesel exhaust particles (also known as TRAP).[1] Common molecules in diesel exhaust particles are polyaromatic hydrocarbons, including phenanthrenes, fluorenes, naphthalenes, fluoranthrenes, and pyrenes.[61] They can be very difficult to measure, given their heterogeneity but are associated with IgE and cytokine production, with potential effects on T cells, mast cells, epithelial cells, and macrophages.[54,61] Sulfuric acid is a form of PM and controlled studies using it have shown a decreased FEV_1 during exercise in asthma patients.[58] Increases of over 10 µg/m^3 in PM_{10} have been associated with increased emergency department asthma visits.[58] Even PM concentrations of less than 10 µg/m^3 annual mean are associated with increased asthma incidence.[62] Diesel exhaust particulate exposure has been linked to an increase in methacholine responsiveness within 24 hours of exposure.[63]

Lipopolysaccharides

Lipopolysaccharide (LPS) or endotoxin has been found in PM, and this has been shown to cause airway inflammation (predominantly neutrophils) in bronchial challenges.[54] Patients with allergic asthma can thus be more affected by exposure to LPS.[54]

Clinical effects of air pollution

Older asthma patients may be more susceptible to a reduction in lung function and increased hospital admissions due to PM$_{2.5}$, ozone, and nitrogen dioxide.[64] One study in the greater Cincinnati area showed mean daily residential exposure to traffic exhaust was linked to worse asthma symptom control of older adults.[64]

Children with asthma are thought to be at risk from air pollution adverse effects due to developing lungs, increased ventilation rates, and developing metabolism.[1] Increased symptoms and medication use have been associated with PM air pollution in children in southern California.[58] Another study from California demonstrated that hospital visits for asthma are associated with local air pollution, especially with girls and infants.[65] One study in the Seattle, WA, area found increases in PM$_{2.5}$ and PM$_{10}$ accompanied greater risks of asthma medication use and asthma exacerbations.[66] International studies have shown similar associations.[67,68] However, there is no certain evidence that air pollution is implicated in the actual development of asthma.[58]

Prevention

Asthma patients should live at a distance of at least 300 m from major traffic roadways.[1] Local communities and governments should issue pollution alerts on days when PM or ozone levels are elevated.[1] On days of high pollution, asthma patients should ideally stay indoors and avoid prolonged outdoor air exposure.[1] Finding alternative commuting routes away from major roadways can also be beneficial.[63] Policy issues worldwide should work to reduce the production of air pollutants.[1]

THE IMPACT OF AIR POLLUTANTS ON EPITHELIAL BARRIERS IN ALLERGIC DISEASE STRUCTURE

The epithelium functions as a protective barrier for many organ systems including the skin, nose, lungs, and gastrointestinal tract.[69] Epithelial barriers are very complex structures composed of tight junctions (TJs) that form an apical junctional complex (AJC) surrounding the apicolateral region, apical junctions located underneath the TJs that regulate the apical-basolateral membrane structure and desmosomes, located on the lateral surface of the epithelial cells, which connect the epithelial cells (**Fig. 1**).[69] Epithelial cells are polarized consisting of membrane-bound lipids and proteins and their polarity partly depends on the formation of cell–cell junctions that comprise the AJC.[69] Adherens junctions and TJs are continuously undergoing

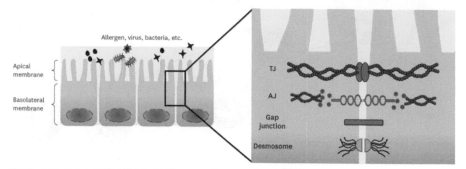

Fig. 1. Structure of the epithelial barrier. (*From* Leland EM, Zhang Z, Kelly KM, Ramanathan M Jr. Role of Environmental Air Pollution in Chronic Rhinosinusitis. *Curr Allergy Asthma Rep.* 2021;21(8):42. Published 2021 Sep 9.)

turnover and recycling (see **Fig. 1**).[69] The cytosolic side of the AJC is made-up of structural proteins and their assembly and disassembly regulate epithelial cell shape and differentiation.[69] TJs act as boundaries between apical and basolateral domains of the AJC and act as semipermeable barriers important for transport of ions, solutes, and water.[69] Thus, TJs are critical for formation of epithelial and endothelial cell sheets that form the structural walls and barriers of skin, blood vessels, and body organs that are important for protecting the host from external threats such as allergens, air pollutants, and infectious agents and for maintaining homeostasis.[69] The structural components of transmembrane junctional components are discussed in greater detail elsewhere.[69,70]

Immunopathogenesis of the Epithelial Barrier

There is a complex interaction between the epithelium, environmental determinants, and the immune system. Epithelial cells secrete the cytokines, IL-25, IL-33, and thymic stromal lymphopoietin (TSLP), called alarmins in response to several allergic and nonallergic triggers. These cytokines activate dendritic cells and Group 2 innate lymphoid cells (ILC2s), which produce IL-4, IL-5, IL-9, and IL-13 and other effector molecules that lead to a Th2 immune response (**Fig. 2**).[71,72] It has also been reported that ILC2s may disrupt the epithelial barrier through IL-13.[73]

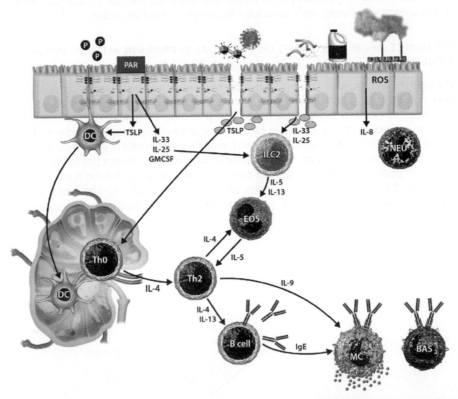

Fig. 2. Epithelial cell activation leading to type 2 inflammation. (*From* Celebi Sözener Z, Cevhertas L, Nadeau K, Akdis M, Akdis CA. Environmental factors in epithelial barrier dysfunction. *J Allergy Clin Immunol.* 2020;145(6):1517-1528.)

Table 1
Environmental factors and mechanisms for disruption of the epithelium[69]

Environmental Factor	Mechanism
Protease allergens	• Elicit non-IgE-mediated reactions via proteinase-activated receptors • Degrade barrier proteins • Increase epithelial permeability
Detergents	• Impair lipid–lipid, lipid–protein interactions of stratum corneum • Disrupt TJs by cleaving occludin and ZO-1 • Increase paracellular permeability • Induce Th2 response by increasing IL-33 and TSLP
Cigarettes and E-cigarettes	• Increase alveolar epithelial permeability • Decrease the level of TJ and AJ proteins • Impact the adhesive intercellular junctions • Disrupt monolayer integrity • Destabilize cell adhesion • Cause worse alveolar fluid clearance
Ozone	• Cause cell stress, desquamation, and death through ROS • Increase protein leakage, and neutrophil and macrophage influx • Induce IL-1α and IL-33 production from epithelial and myeloid cells • Alter cell junction proteins • Increase peribronchial collagen deposition • Chronic exposure cause remodeling, fibrosis, and emphysema
$PM_{2.5}$, PM_{10}, diesel exhaust	• Damage TJ proteins such as occludin, claudin-1, and ZO-1 • Downregulate claudin-1 expression in human airway cells • $PM_{2.5}$ suppresses the levels of E-cadherin (in a mouse model) • PM_{10} and diesel exhaust particles cause reduction and dissociation in occludin from ZO-1 • Increase ROS in the epithelium • Loss of cytokeratin, filaggrin, and E-cadherin
NPs	• Have strong affinity to lipids • Wrap themselves within epithelial membranes • Disrupt cell membrane integrity • Increase paracellular permeability • Induce ROS • Induce cell death (apoptosis, pyroptosis, necrosis)
Microplastic	• Aid in lipid movement in the lipid bilayer • Changes the structure of cell membranes • Because of their 3-dimensional structure they are internalized by cells • Induce proapoptotic protein expression • Alter metabolic profile of bronchial epithelial cells • Cause oxidative stress

Abbreviation: ZO-1, zonula occludens -1.
PM_{10}, PM with diameter <2.5 μm.
Adapted from Celebi Sözener Z, Cevhertas L, Nadeau K, Akdis M, Akdis CA. Environmental factors in epithelial barrier dysfunction. *J Allergy Clin Immunol.* 2020;145(6):1517-1528.

Health Effects of Air Pollutants on a Disrupted Epithelium

Disruption of the epithelium leads to a permeable epithelium causing dysbiosis which is an imbalance in the microflora that can induce tissue inflammation.[74] Changes in the microbiome are now recognized as being important for shaping the immune system and tissue homeostasis of different organ systems including the upper and lower respiratory tracts and gastrointestinal tract (see **Fig. 2**).[70,74] In general, when the host is exposed to chemical irritants, pollutants or protease allergens, non-IgE-mediated reactions occur through activation of protease-activated receptors (ie, protease-activated receptor 2) causing epithelial cells to release alarmins such as TSLP, which induces an innate immune response leading airway inflammation (see **Fig. 2**).[69] This response can also facilitate allergen presentation to the immune system, thereby increasing allergic sensitization leading to secondary inflammatory reactions.

Studies have investigated the health effects of PM, ozone, diesel exhaust, cVOCs emitted from cleaning products, nanoparticles, and microplastics (**Table 1**).[69] PM has been the best characterized, and there are many potential mechanisms for the effect of these pollutants on the epithelium leading to inflammatory changes such as gene transcription, cytokine production, and macrophage polarization.[69] In a model using human nasal epithelial cells, PM has been previously demonstrated to disrupt the TJ leading to increased cytotoxicity due to the release of cytokines (ie, Tumor necrosis factor [TNF]-α, IL-1β, and IL-6) and several micro-RNAs (miRNAs) (ie, MiR-19a and MiR-614) that target the 3'-untranslated region (UTR) of retinoic acid-related orphan receptor alpha (RORα) important for inhibiting inflammation.[75] Air pollutants (ie, PM, O_3, and diesel exhaust particulate) also result in increased production of reactive oxygen species (ROS) that can damage deoxyribonucleic acid (DNA), lipids, and proteins resulting in the production of increased inflammatory cytokines that can increase recruitment of inflammatory cells such as neutrophils, macrophages, monocytes to different organ systems including the nasal cavity and lung, leading to chronic rhinitis and asthma, respectively.[69,70,75]

SUMMARY

Air pollutants are well-known to disrupt the epithelium leading to specific diseases in any organ system that has epithelial linings. The nose and lung are direct targets of respirable air pollutants. Over the last two decades, the discovery of alarmins released by epithelial cells has resulted in a better understanding of the pathogenesis of inflammatory responses associated with allergic and non-AR and asthma. This has led to the recent development of novel biologics that block TSLP, IL-25, and IL-33, culminating with the recent Food Drug Administration (FDA) approval of an anti-TSLP monoclonal antibody for the treatment of asthma.[76–78] Based on our current understanding of the health effects of air pollutants, the charge of the allergist/immunologist should be to advise their patients on avoiding irritant exposures that could damage the epithelial layer in the upper and lower respiratory tracts. On a broader scale, it is our responsibility to advocate for realistic environmental legislation that can achieve necessary standards for improving outdoor and indoor air quality that will favorably impact societal health and prevent disease.

CLINICS CARE POINTS

- Studies suggest that the establishment of the immune response after exposure to air pollutants vary depending on the subject population studied, their socioeconomic status, the respiratory organ affected, and the specific pollutant studied. It is for these reasons that data establishing a relationship between AR and air pollution are variable and often inconsistent.

- The prevalence of allergic rhinitis induced by environmental pollutants in children and adults is poorly elucidated likely due to methodologic differences in epidemiological study design and exposure assessment methods including exposure duration. However, a recent systematic review and meta-analysis found that the effect of air pollutants on allergic rhinitis (AR), except for particulate matter (PM_{10}), was significant and higher in developing countries than in developed countries.

- Asthma patients should live at a distance of at least 300 m from major traffic roadways. Local communities and governments should issue pollution alerts on days when PM or ozone levels are elevated. On days of high pollution, asthma patients should ideally stay indoors and avoid prolonged outdoor air exposure. Finding alternative commuting routes away from major roadways can also be beneficial. Policy issues worldwide should work to reduce the production of air pollutants.

- Air pollutants disrupt the epithelium leading to specific diseases involving the nose and lung. The discovery of alarmins, TSLP, IL-25, and IL-33, released by epithelial cells has resulted in a better understanding of the pathogenesis of inflammatory responses associated with allergic and nonallergic rhinitis and asthma culminating with the recent FDA approval of an anti-TSLP monoclonal antibody for the treatment of asthma.

CONFLICTS OF INTEREST

A. Nanda: None.

S.S. Mustafa: Genentech, Regeneron/Sanofi, GSK, AstraZeneca, CSL Behring, Aimmune.

M. Castillo: None.

J.A. Bernstein: INEOS; Speaking: Sanofi-Regeneron, AZ, GSK, Novartis, Genentech, Takeda/Shire, CSL Behring, Biocryst, Pharming, Optinose; Research and consultant: Sanofi-Regeneron, AZ, GSK, Novartis, Genentech, Takeda/Shire, CSL Behring, Biocryst, Pharming, Kalvista, IONIS, Celldex, TLL, ONO, Escient, Cycle, Blueprint Medicine, Biomarin, Merck, Amgen.

REFERENCES

1. Guarnieri M, Balmes JR. Outdoor air pollution and asthma. Lancet 2014;383: 1581–92.
2. Hamidou Soumana I, Carlsten C. Air pollution and the respiratory microbiome. J Allergy Clin Immunol 2021;148:67–9.
3. Li CH, Sayeau K, Ellis AK. Air pollution and allergic rhinitis: role in symptom exacerbation and strategies for management. J Asthma Allergy 2020;13:285–92.
4. Perez L, Declercq C, Iniguez C, et al. Chronic burden of near-roadway traffic pollution in 10 European cities (APHEKOM network). Eur Respir J 2013;42: 594–605.
5. Wu R, Guo Q, Fan J, et al. Association between air pollution and outpatient visits for allergic rhinitis: Effect modification by ambient temperature and relative humidity. Sci Total Environ 2022;821:152960.
6. Pacheco SE, Guidos-Fogelbach G, Annesi-Maesano I, et al. Climate change and global issues in allergy and immunology. J Allergy Clin Immunol 2021;148: 1366–77.

7. United Nations Framework Convention on Climate Change. 1992. Available at: https://unfccc.int/files/essential_background/background_publications_htmlpdf/application/pdf/conveng.pdf. Accessed June 6, 2021.

8. World Health Organization. Air Pollution. 2021. Available at: https://www.who.int/health-topics/air-pollution#tab5tab_1. Accessed June 28, 2021.

9. Cohen AJ, Brauer M, Burnett R, et al. Estimates and 25-year trends of the global burden of disease attributable to ambient air pollution: an analysis of data from the Global Burden of Diseases Study 2015. Lancet 2017;389:1907–18.

10. Domingo JL, Rovira J. Effects of air pollutants on the transmission and severity of respiratory viral infections. Environ Res 2020;187:109650.

11. Li Y, Mu Z, Wang H, et al. The role of particulate matters on methylation of IFN-gamma and IL-4 promoter genes in pediatric allergic rhinitis. Oncotarget 2018; 9:17406–19.

12. Urrutia-Pereira M, Mello-da-Silva CA, Sole D. COVID-19 and air pollution: a dangerous association? Allergol Immunopathol (Madr) 2020;48:496–9.

13. Raulf M, Buters J, Chapman M, et al. Monitoring of occupational and environmental aeroallergens– EAACI position paper. Concerted action of the EAACI IG occupational allergy and aerobiology & air pollution. Allergy 2014;69:1280–99.

14. Poole JA, Barnes CS, Demain JG, et al. Impact of weather and climate change with indoor and outdoor air quality in asthma: a work group report of the AAAAI environmental exposure and respiratory health committee. J Allergy Clin Immunol 2019;143:1702–10.

15. Ziska LH, Gebhard DE, Frenz DA, et al. Cities as harbingers of climate change: common ragweed, urbanization, and public health. J Allergy Clin Immunol 2003; 111:290–5.

16. Beck I, Jochner S, Gilles S, et al. High environmental ozone levels lead to enhanced allergenicity of birch pollen. PLoS One 2013;8:e80147.

17. Reinmuth-Selzle K, Kampf CJ, Lucas K, et al. Air pollution and climate change effects on allergies in the anthropocene: abundance, interaction, and modification of allergens and adjuvants. Environ Sci Technol 2017;51:4119–41.

18. D'Amato G, Cecchi L, D'Amato M, et al. Climate change and respiratory diseases. Eur Respir Rev 2014;23:161–9.

19. Traidl-Hoffmann C, Kasche A, Menzel A, et al. Impact of pollen on human health: more than allergen carriers? Int Arch Allergy Immunol 2003;131:1–13.

20. Sharma KI, Abraham R, Mowrey W, et al. The association between pollutant levels and asthma-related emergency department visits in the bronx after the world trade center attacks. J Asthma 2019;56:1049–55.

21. Eguiluz-Gracia I, Mathioudakis AG, Bartel S, et al. The need for clean air: the way air pollution and climate change affect allergic rhinitis and asthma. Allergy 2020; 75:2170–84.

22. Hehua Z, Qing C, Shanyan G, et al. The impact of prenatal exposure to air pollution on childhood wheezing and asthma: a systematic review. Environ Res 2017; 159:519–30.

23. Li S, Wu W, Wang G, et al. Association between exposure to air pollution and risk of allergic rhinitis: a systematic review and meta-analysis. Environ Res 2022;205: 112472.

24. Papadopoulos NG, Bernstein JA, Demoly P, et al. Phenotypes and endotypes of rhinitis and their impact on management: a PRACTALL report. Allergy 2015;70: 474–94.

25. Naclerio R, Ansotegui IJ, Bousquet J, et al. International expert consensus on the management of allergic rhinitis (AR) aggravated by air pollutants: Impact of air

pollution on patients with AR: current knowledge and future strategies. World Allergy Organ J 2020;13:100106.

26. Chen CC, Chiu HF, Yang CY. Air pollution exposure and daily clinical visits for allergic rhinitis in a subtropical city: Taipei, Taiwan. J Toxicol Environ Health A 2016;79:494–501.

27. Juskiene I, Prokopciuk N, Franck U, et al. Indoor air pollution effects on pediatric asthma are submicron aerosol particle-dependent. Eur J Pediatr 2022;181: 2469–80.

28. Hassoun Y, James C, Bernstein DI. The effects of air pollution on the development of atopic disease. Clin Rev Allergy Immunol 2019;57:403–14.

29. Anderson JO, Thundiyil JG, Stolbach A. Clearing the air: a review of the effects of particulate matter air pollution on human health. J Med Toxicol 2012;8:166–75.

30. Saxena A, Shekhawat S. Ambient air quality classification by grey wolf optimizer based support vector machine. J Environ Public Health 2017;2017:3131083.

31. Brugha R, Grigg J. Urban air pollution and respiratory infections. Paediatr Respir Rev 2014;15:194–9.

32. Li N, Georas S, Alexis N, et al. A work group report on ultrafine particles (American Academy of Allergy, Asthma & Immunology): why ambient ultrafine and engineered nanoparticles should receive special attention for possible adverse health outcomes in human subjects. J Allergy Clin Immunol 2016;138:386–96.

33. Lennon S, Zhang Z, Lessmann R, et al. Experiments on particle deposition in the human upper respiratory system. Aerosol Sci Technol 2007;28:464–74.

34. Gehring U, Gruzieva O, Agius RM, et al. Air pollution exposure and lung function in children: the ESCAPE project. Environ Health Perspect 2013;121:1357–64.

35. Burte E, Leynaert B, Bono R, et al. Association between air pollution and rhinitis incidence in two European cohorts. Environ Int 2018;115:257–66.

36. Deng Q, Lu C, Yu Y, et al. Early life exposure to traffic-related air pollution and allergic rhinitis in preschool children. Respir Med 2016;121:67–73.

37. Maio S, Baldacci S, Carrozzi L, et al. Respiratory symptoms/diseases prevalence is still increasing: a 25-yr population study. Respir Med 2016;110:58–65.

38. Borlee F, Yzermans CJ, Aalders B, et al. Air pollution from livestock farms is associated with airway obstruction in neighboring residents. Am J Respir Crit Care Med 2017;196:1152–61.

39. Rosario Filho NA, Urrutia-Pereira M, D'Amato G, et al. Air pollution and indoor settings. World Allergy Organ J 2021;14:100499.

40. Logue JM, Klepeis NE, Lobscheid AB, et al. Pollutant exposures from natural gas cooking burners: a simulation-based assessment for Southern California. Environ Health Perspect 2014;122:43–50.

41. Breysse PN, Diette GB, Matsui EC, et al. Indoor air pollution and asthma in children. Proc Am Thorac Soc 2010;7:102–6.

42. Gillespie-Bennett J, Pierse N, Wickens K, et al. The respiratory health effects of nitrogen dioxide in children with asthma. Eur Respir J 2011;38:303–9.

43. Nurmatov UB, Tagiyeva N, Semple S, et al. Volatile organic compounds and risk of asthma and allergy: a systematic review. Eur Respir Rev 2015;24:92–101.

44. Kurmi OP, Lam KB, Ayres JG. Indoor air pollution and the lung in low- and medium-income countries. Eur Respir J 2012;40:239–54.

45. Ruggieri S, Drago G, Longo V, et al. Sensitization to dust mite defines different phenotypes of asthma: A multicenter study. Pediatr Allergy Immunol 2017;28: 675–82.

46. Platts-Mills TA. The allergy epidemics: 1870-2010. J Allergy Clin Immunol 2015; 136:3–13.

47. Katelaris CH, Beggs PJ. Climate change: allergens and allergic diseases. Intern Med J 2018;48:129–34.

48. Thacher JD, Gruzieva O, Pershagen G, et al. Mold and dampness exposure and allergic outcomes from birth to adolescence: data from the BAMSE cohort. Allergy 2017;72:967–74.

49. Mitamura Y, Nunomura S, Nanri Y, et al. The IL-13/periostin/IL-24 pathway causes epidermal barrier dysfunction in allergic skin inflammation. Allergy 2018;73:1881–91.

50. de Brito JM, Mauad T, Cavalheiro GF, et al. Acute exposure to diesel and sewage biodiesel exhaust causes pulmonary and systemic inflammation in mice. Sci Total Environ 2018;628-629:1223–33.

51. Rider CF, Yamamoto M, Gunther OP, et al. Controlled diesel exhaust and allergen coexposure modulates microRNA and gene expression in humans: Effects on inflammatory lung markers. J Allergy Clin Immunol 2016;138:1690–700.

52. Liu Y, Pan J, Zhang H, et al. Short-Term Exposure to Ambient Air Pollution and Asthma Mortality. Am J Respir Crit Care Med 2019;200:24–32.

53. Gilliland FD, Li YF, Saxon A, et al. Effect of glutathione-S-transferase M1 and P1 genotypes on xenobiotic enhancement of allergic responses: randomised, placebo-controlled crossover study. Lancet 2004;363:119–25.

54. Peden DB. Air pollution in asthma: effect of pollutants on airway inflammation. Ann Allergy Asthma Immunol 2001;87:12–7.

55. Goodman JE, Zu K, Loftus CT, et al. Short-term ozone exposure and asthma severity: Weight-of-evidence analysis. Environ Res 2018;160:391–7.

56. Jerrett M, Burnett RT, Pope CA 3rd, et al. Long-term ozone exposure and mortality. N Engl J Med 2009;360:1085–95.

57. Cifuentes L, Borja-Aburto VH, Gouveia N, et al. Assessing the health benefits of urban air pollution reductions associated with climate change mitigation (2000-2020): Santiago, Sao Paulo, Mexico City, and New York City. Environ Health Perspect 2001;109(Suppl 3):419–25.

58. Koenig JQ. Air pollution and asthma. J Allergy Clin Immunol 1999;104:717–22.

59. Zheng XY, Orellano P, Lin HL, et al. Short-term exposure to ozone, nitrogen dioxide, and sulphur dioxide and emergency department visits and hospital admissions due to asthma: a systematic review and meta-analysis. Environ Int 2021;150:106435.

60. Barnes PJ. Air pollution and asthma. Postgrad Med J 1994;70:319–25.

61. Peterson B, Saxon A. Global increases in allergic respiratory disease: the possible role of diesel exhaust particles. Ann Allergy Asthma Immunol 1996;77:263–8 [quiz: 9-70].

62. Schiavoni G, D'Amato G, Afferni C. The dangerous liaison between pollens and pollution in respiratory allergy. Ann Allergy Asthma Immunol 2017;118:269–75.

63. North ML, Alexis NE, Ellis AK, et al. Air pollution and asthma: how can a public health concern inform the care of individual patients? Ann Allergy Asthma Immunol 2014;113:343–6.

64. Epstein TG, Ryan PH, LeMasters GK, et al. Poor asthma control and exposure to traffic pollutants and obesity in older adults. Ann Allergy Asthma Immunol 2012;108:423–428 e2.

65. Delfino RJ, Chang J, Wu J, et al. Repeated hospital encounters for asthma in children and exposure to traffic-related air pollution near the home. Ann Allergy Asthma Immunol 2009;102:138–44.

66. Slaughter JC, Lumley T, Sheppard L, et al. Effects of ambient air pollution on symptom severity and medication use in children with asthma. Ann Allergy Asthma Immunol 2003;91:346–53.
67. Garty BZ, Kosman E, Ganor E, et al. Emergency room visits of asthmatic children, relation to air pollution, weather, and airborne allergens. Ann Allergy Asthma Immunol 1998;81:563–70.
68. Rios JL, Boechat JL, Sant'Anna CC, et al. Atmospheric pollution and the prevalence of asthma: study among schoolchildren of 2 areas in Rio de Janeiro, Brazil. Ann Allergy Asthma Immunol 2004;92:629–34.
69. Celebi Sozener Z, Cevhertas L, Nadeau K, et al. Environmental factors in epithelial barrier dysfunction. J Allergy Clin Immunol 2020;145:1517–28.
70. Celebi Sozener Z, Ozdel Ozturk B, Cerci P, et al. Epithelial barrier hypothesis: Effect of the external exposome on the microbiome and epithelial barriers in allergic disease. Allergy 2022;77:1418–49.
71. Akdis CA, Arkwright PD, Bruggen MC, et al. Type 2 immunity in the skin and lungs. Allergy 2020;75:1582–605.
72. Pasha MA, Patel G, Hopp R, et al. Role of innate lymphoid cells in allergic diseases. Allergy Asthma Proc 2019;40:138–45.
73. Sugita K, Steer CA, Martinez-Gonzalez I, et al. Type 2 innate lymphoid cells disrupt bronchial epithelial barrier integrity by targeting tight junctions through IL-13 in asthmatic patients. J Allergy Clin Immunol 2018;141:300–310 e11.
74. Xue Y, Chu J, Li Y, et al. The influence of air pollution on respiratory microbiome: a link to respiratory disease. Toxicol Lett 2020;334:14–20.
75. Leland EM, Zhang Z, Kelly KM, et al. Role of environmental air pollution in chronic rhinosinusitis. Curr Allergy Asthma Rep 2021;21:42.
76. Marone G, Spadaro G, Braile M, et al. Tezepelumab: a novel biological therapy for the treatment of severe uncontrolled asthma. Expert Opin Investig Drugs 2019;28:931–40.
77. Matera MG, Rogliani P, Calzetta L, et al. TSLP inhibitors for asthma: current status and future prospects. Drugs 2020;80:449–58.
78. Pelaia C, Pelaia G, Longhini F, et al. Monoclonal antibodies targeting alarmins: a new perspective for biological therapies of severe asthma. Biomedicines 2021;9.

Influence of Rural Environmental Factors in Asthma

Jennilee Luedders, MD*, Jill A. Poole, MD

KEYWORDS

- Rural • Agriculture • Asthma • Wheeze

KEY POINTS

- Rural populations are at risk for unique agriculture-related exposures that likely contribute to worsening asthma and wheeze.
- Exposures to certain pesticides, livestock facilities, agricultural dust, endotoxin (specifically late-life endotoxin exposure), and biomass fuel smoke should be considered as risk factors for asthma and/or wheeze.
- Minimizing exposure to the aforementioned rural risk factors may help reduce negative respiratory effects in agricultural communities and further investigations into these risk factors are warranted.
- Early-life endotoxin exposure and certain dietary factors (particularly omega-3 fatty acids and unpasteurized milk) are potentially protective factors in relation to rural airway inflammation.

INTRODUCTION

When compared with those who live in metropolitan counties, dwellers of rural areas within the United States have increased percentages of preventable deaths from the five leading causes of death (ie, cancer, heart disease, unintentional injury, chronic lower respiratory disease, and stroke), with the largest disparity demonstrated from chronic respiratory disease.[1] It is also recognized that people who reside in rural communities have less access to health care and worse health-related outcomes.[2] There are several barriers to care, which may contribute to health disparities for those in rural communities including transportation issues, cost, language differences, and immigration concerns.[3] In a survey sponsored by the US Department of Labor, it was shown that among farmworkers with asthma, the most commonly reported barriers

Division of Allergy and Immunology, Department of Internal Medicine, College of Medicine, University of Nebraska Medical Center, 985990 Nebraska Medical Center, Omaha, NE 68198, USA
* Corresponding author. 985990 Nebraska Medical Center, Omaha, NE 68198-5990.
E-mail address: jennilee.luedders@unmc.edu

Immunol Allergy Clin N Am 42 (2022) 817–830
https://doi.org/10.1016/j.iac.2022.05.008
0889-8561/22/© 2022 Elsevier Inc. All rights reserved.

immunology.theclinics.com

to health care were transportation (60%) and cost (33%).[4] Pate and colleagues[2] used data from the National Health Interview Survey to investigate factors relating to asthma and found that asthma mortality rates were significantly higher for persons of all ages in areas with a population less than 10,000 at 13.4 per 1 million compared with 8.8 per 1 million in large metropolitan areas.

Rural environmental exposures and agriculture-related work are known to be associated with asthma, both occupational (asthma caused by work) and work-exacerbated (preexisting asthma that is aggravated at work).[5] Several studies have suggested that certain farming-related exposures as an adult increase the risk of asthma or asthma-like symptoms development, which contrasts with the hygiene hypothesis concept that suggests that farming and associated microbial exposures are protective against allergic asthma.[5,6] Farmworkers are exposed to a complex working environment with associated disease outcomes dependent on the interplay of many factors including genetics, gender, history of atopy, duration of exposures, livestock, diet, and pesticide exposures.[6,7]

The aim of this article is to review data from the past 5 years pertinent to asthma in rural populations and associated rural risk factors for asthma. PubMed, Embase, and Cumulative Index to Nursing and Allied Health Literature (CINAHL) literature searches were conducted with the assistance of a librarian. Terms searched were rural population, rural health, small town, farming, agriculture, environmental pollution, biomass, pesticides, pollution, asthma, pulmonary disease, chronic obstructive pulmonary disease (COPD), chronic airflow obstruction, and adult. Years searched were 2016 to 2021 and only studies written in English were used. Articles were selected for inclusion after the literature search based on topic fit by author review.

RURAL PESTICIDE EXPOSURE AND IMPACTS ON ASTHMA

There is expanding evidence that suggests that pesticide exposures contribute to allergic and nonallergic asthma and wheeze[8] (**Table 1**). Agricultural workers can be exposed to pesticides via direct inhalation (during spraying or mixing) or via pesticide-contaminated dust.[9] Hoppin and colleagues[8] conducted a comprehensive investigation of the association of pesticides in relationship to wheeze using data from the Agricultural Health Study of male pesticide applicators in North Carolina and Iowa. Associations between pesticide use of 78 different pesticides and wheeze, both allergic (defined as physician-diagnosed hay fever and presence of wheeze) and nonallergic (reporting wheeze but no hay fever), were performed.[8] Of the 78 pesticides examined, 51 had not been previously investigated in relation to respiratory health outcomes.[8] Of greater than 22,000 male pesticide applicator participants, 6% were found to have allergic wheeze and 18% had nonallergic wheeze.[8]

Several of these pesticides ($N = 29$) were positively associated with wheeze including nonallergic wheeze ($N = 21$), allergic wheeze ($N = 19$), and both allergic and nonallergic wheeze ($N = 11$).[8] Seven pesticides had significant ($P < .05$) associations with allergic wheeze versus nonallergic wheeze, including 2,4-D and simazine (herbicides), carbaryl, dimethoate, and zeta-cypermethrin (insecticides).[8] Of the herbicides, 18 of the 43 examined were associated with a wheeze outcome.[8] Clomazone was the only herbicide inversely associated with wheeze (both allergic and nonallergic).[8] Of those positively associated with wheeze, 14 were associated with nonallergic wheeze and 10 were associated with allergic wheeze.[8] The most popularly used herbicides associated with allergic and nonallergic wheeze included glyphosate (trade name Roundup) and atrazine, whereas 2,4-D was associated only with allergic wheeze.[8] Of the insecticides, 9 of the 25 examined were positively associated with

Table 1
Studies investigating pesticides and asthma and/or wheeze from 2016 to 2021

	Pesticide Category					
	Carbamate	**Phenoxy**	**Pyrethroid**	**Organo-chlorine**	**Glyphosate**[a]	**Malathion**[a]
Cherry et al,[9] 2018	No association with asthma	Positive association with asthma	No association with asthma	No association with asthma	Not investigated	No association with asthma
Hoppin et al,[8] 2017	Positive association with wheeze	Positive association with wheeze	Positive association with wheeze	No association with wheeze	Positive association with wheeze	Positive association with wheeze
Patel et al,[11] 2018	Positive association of insecticides with asthma	No association with asthma	Positive association of insecticides with asthma	Not investigated	No association with asthma	Positive association of insecticides with asthma

[a] Types of organophosphorus herbicide.

wheeze.[8] Disulfoton was the only insecticide inversely associated with a wheeze (nonallergic).[8] Malathion, permethrin, and pyrethrins were associated with both allergic and nonallergic wheeze.[8] Carbaryl, chlorpyrifos, dimethoate, and zeta cypermethrin were associated with allergic wheeze, whereas cyfluthrin and Fly Spray were positively associated with nonallergic wheeze.[8] Six fungicides, one fumigant, and one rodenticide were evaluated for association with wheeze and only the rodenticide warfarin was associated with wheeze (allergic).[8] Although nonallergic wheeze was found to be three times as common as allergic wheeze, pesticide associations were stronger with allergic wheeze, potentially implying that pesticides have greater effects in atopic individuals.[8]

In addition, Mazurek and Henneberger[10] showed greater effects of pesticides with allergic asthma versus nonallergic asthma. Using survey data collected from over 11,000 active US farm workers, farmers with allergic rhinitis were 6.03 times more likely to report current asthma and 1.38 times more likely to report exposure to pesticides as compared with farmers without allergic rhinitis. There was also a positive association between pesticide exposure and comorbid asthma and allergic rhinitis.[10] In contrast, the association with pesticides was not significant in those with current asthma without a history of allergic rhinitis.[10]

The Farm and Ranch Safety Survey data from greater than 11,000 farmers[11] also found a relationship between pesticide exposures and asthma. Patel and colleagues[11] showed that insecticide and herbicide use in the last 12 months was associated with current asthma with an adjusted prevalence odds ratio of 1.5 for any pesticide use. It is interesting to note that glyphosate was not shown to have a significant association with current asthma among farmers, which contrasts with the findings from the Agricultural Health Study.[11] The authors hypothesized that this difference could be because of the Agricultural Health Study having a larger number of questions dedicated to pesticide use which could have led to a more thorough assessment of pesticide exposures.[11]

Cherry and colleagues[9] examined the respiratory health of grain farmers exposed to pesticides in Alberta, Canada, to assess pesticide use and respiratory disease and symptoms in greater than 1300 grain farmers. Phenoxy herbicide exposures were associated with self-reported asthma that increased with duration of exposure showing an adjusted odds ratio of 1.29 for 1 to 22 years of exposure, 2.52 for 23 to 34 years of exposure, and 3.18 for greater than 35 years of exposure.[9] After stratification for self-reported allergy, the odds ratios for phenoxy compounds with asthma were higher in those without allergies, suggesting that an irritant mechanism in addition to allergic mechanisms could be considered for this specific pesticide.[9] Thus, it remains unclear if phenoxy compounds induce a form of reactive airways dysfunction syndrome versus allergic-type immune responses.[9]

The mechanisms by which pesticides drive adverse respiratory health consequences remain to be elucidated.[12] To evaluate potential mechanisms, Hoang and colleagues[12] performed an epigenome-wide association study of blood DNA methylation in relation to specific pesticides using the Agricultural Health Study cohort of greater than 1000 farmers of European ancestry. They focused on nine pesticide ingredients for which at least 30 participants had reported past and recent (within the last year) use and seven organochlorines that have been banned.[12] Comparing the methylation at C-phosphate-G sites among those who were exposed to pesticides to those who had never used pesticides, 162 methylated C-phosphate-G sites across eight of the nine pesticide ingredients that are currently available on the market and among one organochlorine were discovered.[12] The differentially methylated C-phosphate-G sites were distinctive for each active ingredient that potentially supports specific methylation patterns for different pesticides.[12] By identifying differential methylation for different pesticide ingredients, this study advances the knowledge of biological mechanisms altered by pesticide exposures.[12]

INFLUENCE OF LIVESTOCK AND ANIMAL PRODUCTION EXPOSURES ON ASTHMA

Livestock exposure in agricultural work settings seems to increase the risk of asthma development and asthma exacerbations as well as COPD.[6] However, it is unclear if asthma symptoms are directly influenced by exposure to the livestock themselves versus influenced by exposure to organic materials (including hay, straw, dust, and animal feed) that are handled when working with livestock.[6] In addition, farmers who work in concentrated animal feeding operations (CAFOS) are exposed to gases, organic dusts, fungal spores, and particulate matter that can all contribute to airway inflammation and obstruction.[5]

Schultz and colleagues[13] performed a study in 2019 to evaluate the association between living in residential communities in close proximity to dairy CAFOs and respiratory health effects within a rural Wisconsin population. Survey data were obtained from 2008 to 2016 of greater than 5000 adults living in rural areas that included distance to nearest CAFO, prevalence of self-reported physician-diagnosed asthma, asthma episodes in the previous 12 months, asthma medication use, allergies, and lung function measured via spirometry.[13] Current asthma was 1.8 to 1.9 times greater in populations living 1 to 3 miles from a CAFO versus those living 5 miles from a CAFO and the odds of having allergies were greater than 2fold when those residing 1 to 1.5 miles from a CAFO were compared with those who lived 5 miles from a CAFO.[13] In addition, when compared with living 5 miles from a CAFO, the odds of ever having received a diagnosis of asthma were 3.11 (95% CI 1.49, 4.36) for those 1 mile from a CAFO and 2.67 (95% CI 1.33, 3.08) for those 1.5 miles from a CAFO.[13] The odds of physician-diagnosed asthma and asthma-related medication use also decreased as the distance from a CAFO increased.[13] Namely, for those within 1, 1.5, 2, and 2.5 miles from a CAFO, asthma medication use was 4, 3, 2.5, and 2 times greater, respectively, relative to the population that lived 5 miles from a CAFO.[13] In addition, the odds of experiencing an asthma attack were 2 times higher for those living 1 to 3 miles versus 5 miles from a CAFO.[13] Correspondingly, lung function measurements were also dependent on proximity to a CAFO as the predicted forced expiratory volume (FEV1) was 7.72% lower when living 1.5 miles from a CAFO as compared with those living 3 miles from a CAFO.[13] In summary, proximity of residence to animal feeding operations may increase the risk for asthma and exacerbate asthma symptoms.

In addition, a case-control study was performed by Rasmussen and colleagues,[14] using electronic health records of a rural Pennsylvania health clinic to investigate residential proximity to swine or dairy/veal industrial food animal productions (IFAP) and the association with asthma exacerbations between groups living less than 3 miles versus those living greater than 3 miles from an IFAP. They found 11% increased odds of oral corticosteroid prescriptions and 29% increased odds of hospitalizations for asthma among the population living within 3 miles of an IFAP when compared with those living greater than 3 miles from an IFAP.[14] These findings are consistent with other studies on IFAP and asthma exacerbations that suggest IFAP as a risk factor for asthma symptoms and reduced lung function.[14–16]

Although asthma was not assessed, a study by Rinsky and colleagues[17] examined associations between animal operations, COPD diagnoses, and respiratory symptoms in more than 22,000 farmers. This study found that raising livestock on medium to large-scale operations was positively associated with chronic bronchitis symptoms, both with and without a history of COPD diagnosis, when compared with farmers who did not raise animals. When comparing specific types of livestock, farmers who raised hogs had increased odds of chronic bronchitis symptoms in groups with a history of COPD (OR 1.41, CI: 1.05–1.89) and without a history of COPD (OR 1.25, CI: 1.06–1.47).[17] In contrast, farmers who raised poultry or beef cattle had increased odds of chronic bronchitis symptoms only in those without a prior diagnosis of COPD (poultry OR 1.29 CI: 0.98–1.70, beef cattle OR 1.29, CI: 0.98–1.70).[17] In farmers with dairy cattle exposure, there was an increased odds of both COPD diagnosis and chronic bronchitis symptoms (OR 1.63, CI: 0.98–2.70).[17] This study suggests that raising livestock is associated with the increase of chronic bronchitis symptoms, but differences in symptoms may be seen among those raising different types of livestock depending on the history of COPD.[17] Future areas of study should consider targeting and investigating these differences as well in association with asthma–COPD overlap (ACO).

RURAL DUST EXPOSURE TO AIRWAY INFLAMMATION

Chronic inhalation of agriculture-related dust has been associated with an increased burden of airway inflammatory diseases including asthma, chronic bronchitis, and COPD.[18] Prior studies have suggested endotoxin, peptidoglycans, components of gram-positive bacterial cell walls, $(1 \rightarrow 3)$-β-D-glucans, and fungi as potential components of dust that may be contributors to the inflammatory response.[18] At this time, there are no known treatments that can reverse respiratory disease induced by complex environmental dust exposures.[19]

To evaluate attributable risk factors for chronic airflow obstruction, including exposure to dusty jobs, the burden of obstructive lung disease study investigated greater than 28,000 participants to determine the prevalence of chronic airway obstruction with various risk factors.[20] Forty-one sites, both rural and urban, across the world were included.[20] Working in a self-reported "dusty job" for greater than 10 years was positively associated with chronic airway obstruction (attributable risk: men: 0.65%; women: 0.29%) of which the highest prevalence for men was in Pakistan (1.6%) and for women was in Austria (0.9%).[20] The limitation of this study is that the "dusty job" exposure was self-reported and thus errors in interpretation could reduce the estimated relative risk and exposures of less than 10 years were not examined.[20]

In a geographically focused study area of rural Colorado prone to dust storms, James and colleagues[21] investigated ambient particulate matter concentrations and the effect on emergency visits, urgent care visits, and hospitalizations (EUH) due to asthma. They showed that for each 15 μg per cubic meter increase in 3-day ambient particulate matter, there was a 3.1% increase in EUH for patients with asthma.[21] In the events when the 3-day average ambient particulate matter exceeded 50 μg per cubic meter, EUH visits increased by 16.8%.[21] Furthermore, when 3-day averages were greater than 100 μg per cubic meter, EUH visits increased by 65.8%.[21] In summary, elevated ambient particulate matter concentrations were associated with increased asthma-associated health care visits in a rural Colorado community prone to dust storms.[21]

The microbiota associated with agriculture exposures and dust also represents an important factor in mediating asthma consequences. For example, Lee and colleagues,[22] sampled dust from bedrooms of homes of farmers and their spouses in North Carolina and Iowa, of which ~55% reported working with crops and ~50% reported working with livestock and collected asthma status data. They showed that the overall diversity of bacteria in house dust was similar between controlled and uncontrolled asthma, but individual taxon types varied.[22] Specifically, taxa from fusobacteria, cyanobacteria, and bacteroidetes were more abundant in the homes of those with uncontrolled asthma, whereas taxa from firmicutes were found to be more prevalent in those with controlled asthma.[22] The phylum firmicutes is known to compose the largest fraction of the gut microbiota and has been previously shown to have a potentially protective association with regard to the degree of asthma control in asthmatics.[23] Dysbiosis, or disruption of microbiota homeostasis, of firmicutes has been associated with respiratory diseases, including asthma.[24]

The identification of the key environmental factors and host defense responses would be advantageous to inform potential novel therapeutic strategies for airway inflammatory diseases encountered in rural environments.[18] To investigate potential treatment targets, Poole and colleagues[19] investigated the role of amphiregulin (AREG), an epidermal growth factor receptor agonist. In the first set of studies, repetitive exposure to swine confinement organic dust extract-induced airway inflammatory consequences that persisted after exposure was removed, and in mice receiving an AREG-neutralizing antibody, this postexposure inflammatory response was increased.[19] Conversely, intranasal administration of recombinant AREG for 3 days post-repetitive exposure was found to hasten the resolution of dust extract-induced inflammatory cell influx and pro-inflammatory cytokine levels within the airway.[19] Mechanistic studies focused on both murine and human lung fibroblasts also showed that the dust extract increased AREG and inflammatory cytokine release as well as inhibited wound closure and recellularization of lung scaffolds.[19] Although these studies suggest that AREG supplementation may be potentially beneficial in improving post-agricultural dust exposure-induced lung disease, additional studies using different rural inflammatory agents (eg, endotoxin, peptidoglycan) and fully characterizing the response over longer time periods are warranted.

Proteases have also been previously implicated in mediating complex agriculture-related organic dust-induced airway inflammation.[25] The potential importance of targeting protease activity in complex dusts was recently investigated by Burr and colleagues,[26] centered on an airborne dust collection near an agricultural drainage reservoir in California called the Salton Sea. The Salton Sea dust extract-induced an inflammatory response in mice that was reduced with protease activity-depleted Salton Sea dust extracts.[26] Correspondingly, the Salton Sea dust extract-induced pro-inflammatory cytokine release from cultured human bronchial epithelial cells, and this response was reduced with protease activity-depleted dust extract as well as in the setting of protease-activated receptor 1 and 2 antagonism.[26]

ENDOTOXIN AND ASTHMA IMPLICATIONS

Endotoxin is a type of lipopolysaccharide present on the outer membrane of gram-negative bacteria that leads to a pro-inflammatory innate immune system response when released as a free lipopolysaccharide.[27] Endotoxin is also found in higher quantities in the dust of homes in rural farming areas when compared with urban or rural nonfarming areas.[28,29] Endotoxin has been previously recognized to play a role in influencing asthma and is associated with inducing asthma exacerbations and COPD.[30–33]

Carnes and colleagues[34] examined the association of house dust endotoxin with asthma and pulmonary function in adults. They performed a case-control study using the Agricultural Health Study to evaluate a population of farmers and farmers' spouses and examined 2485 households with 927 current asthma cases.[34] Dust was collected from the bedrooms of each household, and dust endotoxin levels were measured.[34] In addition, questionnaires, spirometry, and blood draws of the participants were examined.[34] They found that increasing levels of endotoxin were associated with higher odds of current asthma (OR 1.3, CI 1.14–1.47) irrespective of atopy as there were positive associations with both atopic (OR 1.38, CI 1.09–1.74) and nonatopic asthma (OR 1.24, CI 1.07–1.43).[34] In addition, they investigated whether residence on a farm at birth affected the association between asthma and endotoxin.[34] They showed that associations between endotoxin and asthma were significantly higher for those not residing on a farm at birth (OR 1.67, CI 1.26–2.2) when compared with those who were living on a farm at birth (OR 1.18, CI 1.02–1.37).[34] Last, the investigators showed that increasing endotoxin levels were related to lower FEV_1/Forced vital capacity (FVC) in those with asthma (b = 21%, SE = 0.5) when compared with those without asthma (b = 20.05%, SE = 0.2) (interaction P = .01).[34]

In contrast to the former study by Carnes and colleagues showing an increased odds of asthma in adults with endotoxin exposure, a protective response with endotoxin exposure with farming practices in pediatric populations has been described. Stein and colleagues[35] examined populations of children of two distinct farming communities, the Amish of Indiana and the Hutterites of South Dakota who have similar lifestyles (particularly for factors thought to influence asthma) but vast differences in asthma prevalence. The Amish follow traditional farming practices and live on single-family farms, in contrast to the Hutterites who tend to use industrialized agricultural practices and live on large, communal farms.[35] Asthma prevalence in Amish children was 5.2%, whereas in Hutterite children, the prevalence was markedly higher at 21.3%.[36,37] Moreover, the prevalence of asthma was 4 times lower in the Amish population, whereas endotoxin levels were 6.8 times higher when compared with those in Hutterite homes.[35] Using a mouse model, intranasal instillation of Amish dust extract before induction of the experimental ovalbumin asthma model led to reduced airway hyperreactivity and eosinophil influx when compared with Hutterite dust extract (P < .001).[35] These responses were dependent on both innate immune MyD88 and Trif signaling pathways.[35] Highlighting the importance of timing of exposure, it has also been shown that exposure to endotoxin-enriched swine confinement organic dust extracts *after* induction of experimental ovalbumin asthma resulted in potentiation (not reduction) of airway inflammatory consequences in mice.[38]

RESPIRATORY EFFECTS OF BIOMASS AND CROP BURNING

The term biomass encompasses recently living plant or animal-based material (including wood, crop residue, and animal waste) that can be burned for fuel purposes[39] and represents an important rural area air pollutant that has been associated with airway inflammatory processes of both asthma and COPD.[40] ACO refers to a heterogeneous entity of chronic respiratory disease with features of both asthma and COPD that tends toward lower quality of life than with either disease alone.[29] Morgan and colleagues[29] investigated risk factors, including biomass fuels, for ACO among adults in various middle- and low-income countries including Peru, Argentina, Chile, Uruguay, Bangladesh, and Uganda. Biomass fuel smoke exposure was associated with higher odds of having ACO (OR 1.48, 95% CI 0.98–2.23) when compared with those without obstruction or asthma, therefore biomass smoke exposure should be considered as a risk factor for ACO development.[29]

Crop burning is another common practice used after harvests to rapidly clear land for shifting cultivation and to remove vegetation to increase agricultural productivity.[41] Prior studies have suggested that crop burning releases air pollutants and has negative impacts on respiratory health.[42] A 2021 study by Rutlen and colleagues[43] examined the effects of crop burning on emergency department treatments for asthma and COPD in rural Arkansas whereby Craighead county burns approximately half of the acres each year following harvest and Sebastian county does not practice crop burning. Emergency room visits were increased by 20.9% for asthma (95% CI 1.01–1.45, $P = .04$) and 16.9% for COPD (95% CI 1.06–1.29, $P = .003$) during the fall months in Craighead county when compared with Sebastian county after controlling for sex, age, and race.[43] Correspondingly, particulate matter (PM) 2.5 concentrations were significantly ($P = .005$) elevated in Craighead county relative to Sebastian county only during the fall season.[43]

PROTECTIVE EFFECTS OF DIET ON PULMONARY INFLAMMATION

Nutrients and dietary components have been considered potentially important factors which may have an impact on chronic lung disease and inflammation.[44,45] To investigate the potential protective effects of diet in those exposed to agricultural dusts, Ulu and colleagues[45] investigated a potential therapeutic role of docosahexaenoic acid (DHA), a polyunsaturated omega-3 fatty acid, in airway inflammation resolution. Mice were fed either a high-DHA diet or a control diet and then exposed to swine confinement dust extract for 3 weeks followed by a 1-week recovery period.[45] Mice in the high-DHA diet group showed improved recovery of airway inflammatory markers evidenced by elevated levels of DHA-derived pro-resolvins and decreased levels of airway inflammatory cells and mediators.[45] This study supports a potential protective role for omega-3 fatty acids in reducing airway inflammatory disease with regard to agricultural dust exposures and suggests that additional future studies are warranted to explore translational approaches.[45]

Wyss and colleagues[7] examined the effect of consumption of raw or unpasteurized milk practices of children within the Agricultural Lung Health Study. They showed that those who consumed raw milk had higher FEV_1 ($\beta = 49.5$ mL, 95% CI 2.8–96.1 mL, $P = .04$) and FVC ($\beta = 66.2$ mL, 95% CI 13.2–119.1 mL, $P = .01$) but not FEV_1/FVC ratio ($\beta = 0.4\%$, 95% CI -0.4%–1.1%, $P = .33$) as compared with those who did not consume raw milk.[7] Of those who had consumed raw milk as a child, 91% no longer consumed raw milk and only 7.5% had consumed any raw milk within the last 10 years.[7] After accounting for those who had consumed raw milk in the last 10 years, the associations were not affected.[7] This study implies that early-life raw milk consumption is associated with higher pulmonary function in adulthood, but the explanation for these findings remains unknown.[7] Potential mechanisms suggested by the authors may be related to fat content, microorganism presence, and interferon γ levels.[7]

IMPLICATIONS OF SEX DIFFERENCES ON RURAL AIRWAY DISEASE

Sex differences represent an additional variable that is likely important in the understanding of airway inflammatory disease consequences associated with rural exposures as women may be underrepresented in studies.[46] To explore these associations in asthma, Arroyo and colleagues[4] used the National Agricultural Workers Survey of US hired crop workers. It is interesting to note that women in this study were more likely to report lifetime asthma (OR 1.86, CI 1.28–2.72) and recent asthma (OR 2.42, CI 1.62–3.61) when compared with men.[4]

Similarly, Fix and colleagues[46] investigated the A Consortium of Agricultural Cohort Studies (AGRICOH) consortium to examine respiratory disease among farmers and their spouses in 2021. More than 200,000 participants from both crop and livestock farming operations were included from six different continents and 44% of the participants were women.[46] The median prevalence among women for allergic asthma was 5.5% and nonallergic asthma was 3.5%, whereas the median prevalence among men for both allergic and nonallergic asthma was 3.6%.[46] Moreover, women had a

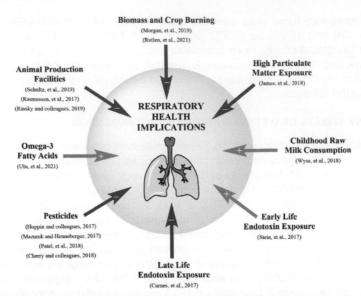

Fig. 1. Rural environmental factors influencing asthma and wheeze. Green arrows represent beneficial influences and red arrows represent detrimental influences. (Figure created with ChemDraw.)

significantly higher prevalence ratio (PR) of allergic asthma to nonallergic asthma in comparison to their male counterparts (PR 0.76, 95% CI 0.72–0.82).[46] Future studies are warranted to understand the increased risk of allergic asthma in women exposed to agricultural risk factors.[46]

SUMMARY

With increased asthma mortality rates shown in rural areas as compared with urban areas,[2] it is increasingly important to develop a more thorough understanding of the environmental risk factors impacting asthma in rural populations and the underlying mechanisms driving airway inflammatory disease. There is a complex network of factors that have potentially significant negative implications on the respiratory health of those residing in rural populations. An overview schematic of the beneficial (or protective) influences versus adverse influences is shown (**Fig. 1**). Increased awareness of these factors that include pesticides, livestock and animal production facilities, agricultural dust, endotoxin, and biomass and crop burning may help to limit exposure and decrease the mortality gap that exists in rural populations affected by asthma. In addition, investigations into nutritional factors and novel strategic approaches to either prevent and/or reduce these adverse health consequences in rural populations are warranted.

CLINICS CARE POINTS

- Pesticide exposures likely contribute to both allergic and nonallergic asthma and wheeze, but these exposures seem to have greater effects in atopic individuals. Considerations should be made by those who work and live in agricultural communities to minimize their risk of pesticide exposure.

- Residential proximity to certain livestock facilities may lead to increased risk for asthma, exacerbation in asthma symptoms, and is associated with reduced lung function. However, differences have been observed according to the type of livestock exposure, and further investigations into these differences could be the focus of future studies.

- Chronic exposure to agricultural dust is associated with increased airway inflammation but currently there are no treatments to reverse respiratory disease related to these complex dust exposures. Amphiregulin supplementation has been identified as potentially beneficial in animal modeling studies.

- Endotoxin has been associated with both asthma exacerbations and chronic obstructive pulmonary disease (COPD), noting differences in airway inflammatory effects may be dependent on the timing of exposure.

- Biomass fuel smoke exposure should be considered as a risk factor for asthma–COPD overlap, and crop burning practices associated with increased particulate matter concentrations may contribute to increased airway inflammation.

- Certain dietary factors, particularly omega-3 fatty acids and unpasteurized milk, may be associated with improved pulmonary function but the underlying mechanisms remain unknown and additional studies are warranted.

ACKNOWLEDGMENTS

The authors would like to thank Danielle Westmark, librarian, at the University of Nebraska Medical Center, for her assistance with the literature search used for this review articles.

FUNDING AND DISCLOSURES

J.A. Poole has received funding from the Department of Defense (PR200793), the National Institute for Occupational Safety and Health (U54OH010162 and R01OH012045), and the Central States Center of Agricultural Safety and Health (CS-CASH). J.A. Poole has received research funding from AstraZeneca and clinical research funding from Takeda and GlaxoSmithKline.

REFERENCES

1. Garcia MC, Rossen LM, Bastian B, et al. Potentially excess deaths from the five leading causes of death in metropolitan and nonmetropolitan counties - United States, 2010-2017. MMWR Surveill Summ 2019;68(10):1–11.
2. Pate CA, Zahran HS, Qin X, et al. Asthma Surveillance - United States, 2006-2018. MMWR Surveill Summ 2021;70(5):1–32. Washington, DC: 2002.
3. Hoerster KD, Mayer JA, Gabbard S, et al. Impact of individual-, environmental-, and policy-level factors on health care utilization among US farmworkers. Am J Public Health 2011;101(4):685–92.
4. Arroyo AJC, Robinson LB, Downing NL, et al. Occupational exposures and asthma prevalence among US farmworkers: National Agricultural Workers Survey, 2003-2014. J Allergy Clin Immunol In Pract 2018;6(6):2135–8.e2.
5. Nordgren TM, Bailey KL. Pulmonary health effects of agriculture. Curr Opin Pulm Med 2016;22(2):144–9.
6. Wunschel J, Poole JA. Occupational agriculture organic dust exposure and its relationship to asthma and airway inflammation in adults. J Asthma 2016;53(5): 471–7.

7. Wyss AB, House JS, Hoppin JA, et al. aw milk consumption and other early-life farm exposures and adult pulmonary function in the Agricultural Lung Health Study. Thorax 2018;73(3):279–82.

8. Hoppin JA, Umbach DM, Long S, et al. Pesticides are Associated with Allergic and Non-Allergic Wheeze among Male Farmers. Environ Health Perspect 2017; 125(4):535–43.

9. Cherry N, Beach J, Senthilselvan A, et al. Pesticide use and asthma in Alberta grain farmers. Int J Environ Res Public Health 2018;15(3). https://doi.org/10.3390/ijerph15030526.

10. Mazurek JM, Henneberger PK. Lifetime allergic rhinitis prevalence among US primary farm operators: findings from the 2011 Farm and Ranch Safety survey. Int Arch Occup Environ Health 2017;90(6):507–15.

11. Patel O, Syamlal G, Henneberger PK, et al. Pesticide use, allergic rhinitis, and asthma among US farm operators. J Agromedicine 2018;23(4):327–35.

12. Hoang TT, Qi C, Paul KC, et al. Epigenome-wide dna methylation and pesticide use in the agricultural lung health study. Environ Health Perspect 2021;129(9). https://doi.org/10.1289/EHP8928.

13. Schultz AA, Peppard P, Gangnon RE, et al. Residential proximity to concentrated animal feeding operations and allergic and respiratory disease. Environ Int 2019; 130:104911.

14. Rasmussen SG, Casey JA, Bandeen-Roche K, et al. Proximity to Industrial Food Animal Production and Asthma Exacerbations in Pennsylvania, 2005-2012. Int J Environ Res Public Health 2017;14(4):362.

15. Schinasi L, Horton RA, Guidry VT, et al. Air pollution, lung function, and physical symptoms in communities near concentrated Swine feeding operations. Epidemiology 2011;22(2):208–15.

16. Schulze A, Rommelt H, Ehrenstein V, et al. Effects on pulmonary health of neighboring residents of concentrated animal feeding operations: exposure assessed using optimized estimation technique. Arch Environ Occup Health 2011;66(3): 146–54.

17. Rinsky JL, Richardson DB, Kreiss K, et al. Animal production, insecticide use and self-reported symptoms and diagnoses of COPD, including chronic bronchitis, in the Agricultural Health Study. Environ Int 2019;127:764–72.

18. Poole JA, Romberger DJ. Immunological and inflammatory responses to organic dust in agriculture. Curr Opin Allergy Clin Immunol 2012;12(2):126–32.

19. Poole JA, Nordgren TM, Heires AJ, et al. Amphiregulin modulates murine lung recovery and fibroblast function following exposure to agriculture organic dust. Am J Physiol Lung Cell Mol Physiol 2020;318(1):L180–91.

20. Burney P, Patel J, Minelli C, et al. Prevalence and population attributable risk for chronic airflow obstruction in a large multinational stud. Am J Respir Crit Care Med 2020;203(11):1353–65.

21. James KA, Strand M, Hamer MK, et al. Health services utilization in asthma exacerbations and PM(10) levels in rural colorado. Ann Am Thorac Soc 2018;15(8): 947–54.

22. Lee MK, Wyss AB, Carnes MU, et al. House dust microbiota in relation to adult asthma and atopy in a US farming population. J Allergy Clin Immunol 2021; 147(3):910–20.

23. Ley RE, Peterson DA, Gordon JI. Ecological and evolutionary forces shaping microbial diversity in the human intestine. Cell 2006;124(4):837–48.

24. Trivedi R, Barve K. Gut microbiome a promising target for management of respiratory diseases. Biochem J 2020;477(14):2679–96.

25. Romberger DJ, Heires AJ, Nordgren TM, et al. Proteases in agricultural dust induce lung inflammation through PAR-1 and PAR-2 activation. Am J Physiol Lung Cell Mol Physiol 2015;309(4):L388–99.
26. Burr AC, Velazquez JV, Ulu A, et al. Lung inflammatory response to environmental dust exposure in mice suggests a link to regional respiratory disease risk. J Inflamm Res 2021;14:4035–52.
27. Nijland R, Hofland T, van Strijp JA. Recognition of LPS by TLR4: potential for anti-inflammatory therapies. Drugs 2014;12(7):4260–73.
28. Barnig C, Reboux G, Roussel S, et al. Indoor dust and air concentrations of endotoxin in urban and rural environments. Lett Appl Microbiol 2013;56(3):161–7.
29. Morgan BW, Grigsby MR, Siddharthan T, et al. Epidemiology and risk factors of asthma-chronic obstructive pulmonary disease overlap in low- and middle-income countries. J Allergy Clin Immunol 2019;143(4):1598–606.
30. Kline JN, Cowden JD, Hunninghake GW, et al. Variable airway responsiveness to inhaled lipopolysaccharide. Am J Respir Crit Care Med 1999;160(1):297–303.
31. Yen YC, Yang CY, Wang TN, et al. Household airborne endotoxin associated with asthma and allergy in elementary schoolage children: a case-control study in Kaohsiung, Taiwan. Environ Sci Pollut Res Int 2020;27(16):19502–9.
32. Mendy A, Salo PM, Cohn RD, et al. House dust endotoxin association with chronic bronchitis and emphysema. Environ Health Perspect 2018;126(3): 037007.
33. Thorne PS, Kulhánková K, Yin M, et al. Endotoxin exposure is a risk factor for asthma: the national survey of endotoxin in United States housing. Am J Respir Crit Care Med 2005;172(11):1371–7.
34. Carnes MU, Hoppin JA, Metwali N, et al. House Dust Endotoxin Levels Are Associated with Adult Asthma in a U.S. Farming Population. Ann Am Thorac Soc 2017; 14(3):324–31.
35. Stein MM, Hrusch CL, Gozdz J, et al. Innate Immunity and Asthma Risk in Amish and Hutterite Farm Children. N Engl J Med 2016;375(5):411–21.
36. Holbreich M, Genuneit J, Weber J, et al. Amish children living in northern Indiana have a very low prevalence of allergic sensitization. J Allergy Clin Immunol 2012; 129(6):1671–3.
37. Motika CA, Papachristou C, Abney M, et al. Rising prevalence of asthma is sex-specific in a US farming population. J Allergy Clin Immunol 2011;128(4):774–9.
38. Warren KJ, Dickinson JD, Nelson AJ, et al. Ovalbumin-sensitized mice have altered airway inflammation to agriculture organic dust. Respir Res 2019; 20(1):51.
39. Bruce N, Perez-Padilla R, Albalak R. Indoor air pollution in developing countries: a major environmental and public health challenge. Bull World Health Organ 2000;78(9):1078–92.
40. Balmes JR. Household air pollution from domestic combustion of solid fuels and health. J Allergy Clin Immunol 2019;143(6):1979–87.
41. Cançado JE, Saldiva PH, Pereira LA, et al. The impact of sugar cane-burning emissions on the respiratory system of children and the elderly. Environ Health Perspect 2006;114(5):725–9.
42. Agarwal R, Awasthi A, Singh N, et al. Epidemiological study on healthy subjects affected by agriculture crop-residue burning episodes and its relation with their pulmonary function tests. Int J Environ Health Res 2013;23(4):281–95.
43. Rutlen C, Orloff M, Bates J, et al. Crop burning and the prevalence of asthma and COPD emergency department treatments in a rural Arkansas county. J Asthma 2021;58(3):293–8.

44. Isaak M, Ulu A, Osunde A, et al. Nutritional Factors in Occupational Lung Disease. Curr Allergy Asthma Rep 2021;21(4):24.
45. Ulu A, Burr A, Heires AJ, et al. A high docosahexaenoic acid diet alters lung inflammation and recovery following repetitive exposure to aqueous organic dust extracts. J Nutr Biochem 2021;97:108797.
46. Fix J, Annesi-Maesano I, Baldi I, et al. Gender differences in respiratory health outcomes among farming cohorts around the globe: findings from the AGRICOH consortium. J Agromedicine 2021;26(2):97–108.

UNITED STATES POSTAL SERVICE ®

Statement of Ownership, Management, and Circulation
(All Periodicals Publications Except Requester Publications)

1. Publication Title	2. Publication Number		3. Filing Date
IMMUNOLOGY AND ALLERGY CLINICS OF NORTH AMERICA	006 – 361		9/18/2022

4. Issue Frequency	5. Number of Issues Published Annually	6. Annual Subscription Price
FEB, MAY, AUG, NOV	4	$354.00

7. Complete Mailing Address of Known Office of Publication *(Not printer)* *(Street, city, county, state, and ZIP+4®)*

ELSEVIER INC.
230 Park Avenue, Suite 800
New York, NY 10169

Contact Person
Malathi Samayan

Telephone *(Include area code)*
91-44-4299-4507

8. Complete Mailing Address of Headquarters or General Business Office of Publisher *(Not printer)*

ELSEVIER INC.
230 Park Avenue, Suite 800
New York, NY 10169

9. Full Names and Complete Mailing Addresses of Publisher, Editor, and Managing Editor *(Do not leave blank)*

Publisher *(Name and complete mailing address)*

DOLORES MELONI, ELSEVIER INC.
1600 JOHN F KENNEDY BLVD. SUITE 1800
PHILADELPHIA, PA 19103-2899

Editor *(Name and complete mailing address)*

TAYLOR HAYES, ELSEVIER INC.
1600 JOHN F KENNEDY BLVD. SUITE 1800
PHILADELPHIA, PA 19103-2899

Managing Editor *(Name and complete mailing address)*

PATRICK MANLEY, ELSEVIER INC.
1600 JOHN F KENNEDY BLVD. SUITE 1800
PHILADELPHIA, PA 19103-2899

10. Owner *(Do not leave blank. If the publication is owned by a corporation, give the name and address of the corporation immediately followed by the names and addresses of all stockholders owning or holding 1 percent or more of the total amount of stock. If not owned by a corporation, give the names and addresses of the individual owners. If owned by a partnership or other unincorporated firm, give its name and address as well as those of each individual owner. If the publication is published by a nonprofit organization, give its name and address.)*

Full Name	Complete Mailing Address
WHOLLY OWNED SUBSIDIARY OF REED/ELSEVIER, US HOLDINGS	1600 JOHN F KENNEDY BLVD. SUITE 1800 PHILADELPHIA, PA 19103-2899

11. Known Bondholders, Mortgagees, and Other Security Holders Owning or Holding 1 Percent or More of Total Amount of Bonds, Mortgages, or Other Securities. If none, check box ▶ ☐ None

Full Name	Complete Mailing Address
N/A	

12. Tax Status *(For completion by nonprofit organizations authorized to mail at nonprofit rates)* *(Check one)*
The purpose, function, and nonprofit status of this organization and the exempt status for federal income tax purposes:
☒ Has Not Changed During Preceding 12 Months
☐ Has Changed During Preceding 12 Months *(Publisher must submit explanation of change with this statement)*

PS Form **3526**, July 2014 *[Page 1 of 4 (see instructions page 4)]* PSN: 7530-01-000-9931   PRIVACY NOTICE: See our privacy policy on www.usps.com.

---

13. Publication Title			14. Issue Date for Circulation Data Below
IMMUNOLOGY AND ALLERGY CLINICS OF NORTH AMERICA			MAY 2022

15. Extent and Nature of Circulation			Average No. Copies Each Issue During Preceding 12 Months	No. Copies of Single Issue Published Nearest to Filing Date
a. Total Number of Copies *(Net press run)*			143	128
b. Paid Circulation *(By Mail and Outside the Mail)*	(1)	Mailed Outside-County Paid Subscriptions Stated on PS Form 3541 *(Include paid distribution above nominal rate, advertiser's proof copies, and exchange copies)*	87	78
	(2)	Mailed In-County Paid Subscriptions Stated on PS Form 3541 *(Include paid distribution above nominal rate, advertiser's proof copies, and exchange copies)*	0	0
	(3)	Paid Distribution Outside the Mails Including Sales Through Dealers and Carriers, Street Vendors, Counter Sales, and Other Paid Distribution Outside USPS®	26	21
	(4)	Paid Distribution by Other Classes of Mail Through the USPS *(e.g., First-Class Mail®)*	0	0
c. Total Paid Distribution *(Sum of 15b (1), (2), (3), and (4))*		▶	113	99
d. Free or Nominal Rate Distribution *(By Mail and Outside the Mail)*	(1)	Free or Nominal Rate Outside-County Copies included on PS Form 3541	16	14
	(2)	Free or Nominal Rate In-County Copies Included on PS Form 3541	0	0
	(3)	Free or Nominal Rate Copies Mailed at Other Classes Through the USPS *(e.g., First-Class Mail)*	0	0
	(4)	Free or Nominal Rate Distribution Outside the Mail *(Carriers or other means)*	0	0
e. Total Free or Nominal Rate Distribution *(Sum of 15d (1), (2), (3) and (4))*		▶	16	14
f. Total Distribution *(Sum of 15c and 15e)*		▶	129	113
g. Copies not Distributed *(See Instructions to Publishers #4 (page #3))*		▶	14	15
h. Total *(Sum of 15f and g)*		▶	143	128
i. Percent Paid *(15c divided by 15f times 100)*		▶	87.59%	87.61%

* If you are claiming electronic copies, go to line 16 on page 3. If you are not claiming electronic copies, skip to line 17 on page 3.

PS Form **3526**, July 2014 *(Page 2 of 4)*

16. Electronic Copy Circulation		Average No. Copies Each Issue During Preceding 12 Months	No. Copies of Single Issue Published Nearest to Filing Date
a. Paid Electronic Copies	▶		
b. Total Paid Print Copies (Line 15c) + Paid Electronic Copies (Line 16a)	▶		
c. Total Print Distribution (Line 15f) + Paid Electronic Copies (Line 16a)	▶		
d. Percent Paid (Both Print & Electronic Copies) (16b divided by 16c × 100)	▶		

☒ I certify that 50% of all my distributed copies (electronic and print) are paid above a nominal price.

17. Publication of Statement of Ownership
☒ If the publication is a general publication, publication of this statement is required. Will be printed in the NOVEMBER 2022 issue of this publication.   ☐ Publication not required.

18. Signature and Title of Editor, Publisher, Business Manager, or Owner

Malathi Samayan - Distribution Controller   *Malathi Samayan*   Date 9/18/2022

I certify that all information furnished on this form is true and complete. I understand that anyone who furnishes false or misleading information on this form or who omits material or information requested on the form may be subject to criminal sanctions (including fines and imprisonment) and/or civil sanctions (including civil penalties).

PS Form **3526**, July 2014 *(Page 3 of 4)*   PRIVACY NOTICE: See our privacy policy on www.usps.com.

Moving?

Make sure your subscription moves with you!

To notify us of your new address, find your **Clinics Account Number** (located on your mailing label above your name), and contact customer service at:

Email: journalscustomerservice-usa@elsevier.com

800-654-2452 (subscribers in the U.S. & Canada)
314-447-8871 (subscribers outside of the U.S. & Canada)

Fax number: 314-447-8029

Elsevier Health Sciences Division
Subscription Customer Service
3251 Riverport Lane
Maryland Heights, MO 63043

*To ensure uninterrupted delivery of your subscription, please notify us at least 4 weeks in advance of move.

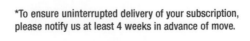

Printed and bound by CPI Group (UK) Ltd, Croydon, CR0 4YY

03/10/2024

01040473-0012